# KETO DIET AFTER 50

*Feel 35 again with this Comprehensive Guide to Ketogenic Diet for Women and Men Over 50. Lose weight and Improve Your Health Easily. Including Exercises, Recipes And a 28-Day Meal Plan*

**Margaret Howell**

# TABLE OF CONTENTS

# Introduction

You are a real champion for deciding on to take charge of your fitness by being more precise about what you eat. And, quite honestly, there are few dietary selections better than keto. However, by sticking with the keto weight loss plan, you are putting your body in the best position to address things like acne, heart diseases, cancer, or even Parkinson's disease.

When you follow the ketogenic diet, you will be able to avoid cravings such as those of sugar and choose something healthier and one that will promote cell development. You will feel fitter, healthier, and sharper.

It is imperative to note that the ketogenic diet for people in their 30s is different from those in their 50s. The main difference is in the amount of energy required to do various activities. In your younger years, you will need more energy to allow you to carry out your activities easily. Weight loss is the most important aspect of a ketogenic diet, and you can easily lose weight with the ketogenic diet. It will help in improving blood sugar levels as well as rejuvenating your brain cells as well as give you a feel-good mood.

# CHAPTER 1:

# Ketogenic Diet Basics

## The Science Behind Keto

There are many scientific theories out there that explain how the human body ages and deteriorates over time, two of which are the free radical theory of aging and glycation theory of aging.

The free radical theory explains that our body becomes damaged because of the free radicals trying to bind to the molecules in our body in their search for more electron, which leads to damage and inflammation. In the process of binding, your molecule becomes unstable and binds with your other molecule to get its electron, and the cycle repeats in a process known as oxidation, causing a lot of damage over time. The proposed solution to this theory is to increase your body's pool of antioxidants because they have an extra electron to give to the free radicals in your body, thus preventing them from taking and destabilizing your body's molecules.

The glycation theory of aging proposes that we age because of the glycation damage from high blood sugar. That means the excess sugar in the body clings onto the proteins in the body, preventing them from doing their jobs, which can lead to many complications, one of which is diabetes.

But how does the keto diet comes in? Keto diets can help the body slow the aging process in many ways: Keto diet minimizes damages done by oxidation and increases the body's store of uric acid and other antioxidants.

Ketosis increases the mitochondrial glutathione, which is a potent antioxidant that resides within the mitochondria, the powerhouse of your cell. Antioxidants that are digested orally are not very effective in protecting your cells. But ketosis supports the cell directly.

Keto diets are very low in sugar, meaning that your blood sugar level would be much lower, reducing the chance of glycation damages.

Keto diets are low in carbs, which improves blood sugar control level and suppress appetite because they have the same effects as fasting.

Keto diets also reduce triglycerides, which are the fatty acids in the bloodstream that are used to measure heart disease risk. You want triglycerides in your body to be as low as possible.

In short, keto diets reduce your blood sugar level, prevent glycation damages, and inflammation. These three conditions are associated with all sorts of diseases that lead to death. Therefore, keto diets ate the best way to reduce blood sugar and insulin levels, increase your longevity and wellbeing.

The carbohydrates that are consumed are converted into glucose and insulin. Here, glucose is sugar. Glucose is the most convenient source of energy because your body can convert it to energy easier. As such, the body prefers using that up first. Another byproduct of carbohydrates is insulin, which is a hormone produced by your pancreas. This hormone helps process glucose in your body by transporting the glucose in the body to where it is needed. When your body has enough energy, the excess glucose will be converted to adipose tissue, or fat, as a backup. Of course, that does not mean that the body uses that fat first if there are carbohydrates available.

You see, the fat in your body is considered to be the backup source of power. Therefore, in a normal situation, your body would burn carbohydrates, then fats, then proteins, in that order. As such, the body does not burn fat as effectively. Ketosis promotes weight loss by making the body prioritize burning fat, thus resulting in more fat being burned.

Many ordinary diets contain plenty of carbohydrates, which are not bad in itself. It is only bad when you take in more energy than you spend it, which means you create an energy leftover which would be converted to fat. Day by day, your weight adds up very quickly. For such a diet, glucose is the main source of energy because it contains plenty of it. However, the glucose in your body can only last you a few days. Your body will convert glucose to fat if you do not use glucose up. So, when your glucose store runs dry in a few days, your body will switch to another source of energy through a biochemical process known as ketogenesis.

When this process starts, your liver starts to take the fat in your body and break it down, creating an alternative source of energy. When that happens, your ketone level goes up and your body. This is the moment when you enter ketosis.

## What is Keto Diet?

Simply, the Keto diet termed a "low-carb" diet burns fuel from fat in the body instead of carbohydrates. It allows you to shed weight efficiently, enjoy an endless source of energy and carves the body into the best state of health both physically and mentally.

Unlike many other low carb diets, you don't stuff yourself with processed foods, unhealthy fried foods (hello Atkins) and all the junk your body craves, which you know are bad for you.

The Keto diet is NOT a hunger strike; you don't need to deprive yourself or limit your food intake in any way. It's about healing your destructive relationship with food, i.e., eating only healthy fun stuff that boosts your self-image and makes you fall in love with exciting food all over again just as you were made to be.

## How does the Keto Diet Work?

On this diet, you strictly reduce your carb intake to allow the body to enter into a state called 'Ketosis.' At this point, the body switches from using carbs but fats to produce energy, and that is where the weight loss magic happens. The lipids are shed!

So, to keep the body pumped with ketones, you ought to ensure a good intake of healthy fats to keep yourself adequately fueled and healthy.

Expect to eat around 70%-80% fat, 25% protein, and 5% carbs. For best results, keep your net carbs under 20g per day (although a more conservative aim would be around 50g)

# Best Foods to Fit into the Keto Diet for Older Adults

## Avocados

Avocados are so famous nowadays in the health community that people associate the word "health" to avocados. This is for a particularly good reason because avocados are extremely healthy. They pack lots of vitamins and minerals such as potassium. Moreover, avocados are shown to help the body go into ketosis faster.

## Berries

Many fruits pack too many carbs that make them unsuitable in a keto diet, but not berries. They are low in carbs and high in fiber. Some of the best berries to include in your diet are blackberries, blueberries, raspberries, and strawberries.

## Butter and Cream

These two food items pack plenty of fat and a very small amount of carbs, making them a good option to include in your keto diet.

## Cheese

Milk is not okay. You can get away with cheese though. Cheese is delicious and nutritious. Thankfully, although there are hundreds of types of cheese out there, all of them are low in carbs and full of fat. Eating cheese may even help your muscles and slow down aging.

## Coconut Oil

Coconut oil and other coconut-related products such as coconut milk and coconut powder are perfect for a keto diet. Coconut oil, especially, contain MCTs that are converted into ketones by the liver to be used as an immediate source of energy.

## Dark Chocolate and Cocoa Powder

These two food items are delicious and contain antioxidants. Dark chocolate is associated with the reduction of heart disease risk by lowering the blood pressure. Just make sure that you choose only dark chocolate with at least 70% cocoa solids.

## Eggs

Eggs form the bulk of most food you will eat in a keto diet because they are the healthiest and most versatile food item of them all. Even a large egg contains so little carbs but packs plenty of protein, making it a perfect option for a keto diet.

Moreover, eggs are shown to have an appetite suppression effect, making you feel full for longer as well as regulating blood sugar levels. This leads to lower calorie intake for about a day. Just make sure to eat the entire egg because the nutrients are in the yolk.

## Meat and Poultry

These two are the staple food in most keto diets. Most of the keto meals revolve around using these two ingredients. This is because they contain no carbs and pack plenty of vitamins and minerals. Moreover, they are a great source of protein.

## Nuts and Seeds

These are also low in carbs but rich in fat. They are also healthy and have a lot of nutrients and fiber. They help reduce heart disease, cancer, depression, and other risks of diseases. The fiber in these also help make you feel full for longer, so you would consume fewer calories and your body would spend more calories digesting them.

## Olive Oil

Olive oil is very beneficial for your heart because it contains oleic acid that helps decrease heart disease risk factors. Extra-virgin olive oil is also rich in antioxidants. The best thing is that olive oil can be used as a main source of fat and it has no carbs. The same goes for olive.

## Plain Greek Yogurt and Cottage Cheese

These two food items are rich in protein and a small number of carbs, small enough that you can safely include them into your keto diet. They also help suppress your appetite by making you feel full for longer and they can be eaten alone and are still delicious.

## Shirataki Noodles

If you love noodles and pasta but don't want to give up on them, then shirataki noodles are the perfect alternative. They are rich in water content and pack a lot of fiber, so that means low carbs and calories and hunger suppression.

## Unsweetened Coffee and Tea

These two drinks are carb-free, so long as you don't add sugar, milk, or any other sweeteners. Both contain caffeine that improves your metabolism and suppresses your appetite. A word of warning to those who love light coffee and tea lattes, though. They are made with non-fat milk and contain a lot of carbs.

## Vegetables

Most vegetables pack a lot of nutrients that your body can greatly benefit from even though they are low in calories and carbs. Plus, some of them contain fiber, which helps with your bowel movement. Moreover, your body spends more energy breaking down and digesting food rich in fiber, so it helps with weight loss as well.

## Meat and Poultry

Chicken, beef, pork, lamb, turkey, veal includes no carb, but high protein and fat intake. That is the primary reason why meat and poultry products are known as the staples for the Ketogenic diet. Besides this, bacon and organ meats are also allowed for consumption.

## Seafood

When it comes to seafood, you also have an excellent list. You can buy and cook a lot of delicious dishes from:

- Lobster

- Mussels

- Octopus

- Oysters

- Salmon

- Scallops

- Shrimp

- Squid

- Tuna

The most useful Keto seafood is the crab and shrimp. They don't contain carbohydrates at all.

## Vegetables

Only low-carb and non-starchy veggies can be eaten by the people who go on the Keto diet. This means that you can add the following vegetables: • Avocados

- Asparagus

- Bell peppers

- Brussel sprouts

- Celery

- Cucumbers

- Eggplant

- Herbs

- Kale

- Kohlrabi

- Lettuce

- Mushrooms

- Mustard

- Radishes

- Spinach

- Tomatoes

- Zucchini

## **Dairy Products**

You should be careful with dairy. Not all dairy food can be useful for you if you want to stick to the Keto diet. Here are the products you can buy and cook: • Butter and ghee

- Cottage cheese

- Eggs

- Hard, semi-hard, soft, and cream cheeses

- Heavy cream and whipping cream

- Sour cream

- Unflavored Greek yogurt

## **Berries**

Unfortunately, most fruits have high levels of carbs and can't be included on the Keto diet. However, you can consume:

- Blackberries

- Blueberries

- Raspberries

- Strawberries

## Nuts and Seeds

A lot of experts recommend paying attention to nuts and seeds that are high-fat and low-carb. You can add such nuts and seeds to your dishes as: • Almond

- Brazil nuts

- Chia seeds

- Flaxseed

- Hazelnuts

- Pecans

- Pumpkin seeds

- Walnuts

• Sesame seeds

## Coconut and Olive Oils

To cook tasty fatty dishes, you need oil. Coconut and olive oils have unique properties that make them suitable for a Keto diet. These oils are rich in fat and boost ketone production. Moreover, they can be used for salad dressing and adding to cooked dishes.

## Low-Carb Drinks

The Keto diet means that you should drink only unsweetened coffee and tea because they don't include carbs and fasten metabolism. Besides, you can drink dark chocolate and cocoa. Such drinks have low levels of carbohydrates and that's why they're permitted.

# Macronutrients of Keto Diet

Unfortunately, one of the main aspects that you will not be able to eat whatever you want when you are following a keto diet. However, like many diets, you will have a wide array of options to choose from. You can find alternatives that you can enjoy and avoid a high carbohydrate diet. The essence of the keto diet is to get your body into ketosis, and all you need to do is to reduce your carbohydrate intake. Carbohydrates are not only the junk foods that you love but also some other healthier foods that you enjoy.

## What Macros Should I Aim for On the Keto Diet After 50?

Macro is a term that is coined from macronutrients, which include protein, fats, and carbohydrates, which makes up the composition of macronutrients required by the body. You can easily find this information listed on the nutritional facts panel of most foods, and you can use counting apps or calculators to calculate your macros. Gram for gram the macronutrients are critical in total calorie count that you will consume per day. One gram of carbohydrate will provide four calories; one gram of protein provides four calories, while one gram of fat will give you nine calories.

Alcohol is also considered a macronutrient, and it gives seven calories per gram, although it has no nutritional value to the body. When you follow your macro diet, you will go beyond counting calories, and you will focus more on macros. Depending on your health objectives, you can adjust the ratios of the macronutrients that you consume to help you build muscle, lose weight, or enter a maintenance mode. If you follow a ketogenic diet, you will pay attention to net carbohydrates as part of the macros because it will determine how many useful carbohydrates you will consume per meal.

The macronutrients mustn't be confused with micronutrients, which are the key vitamins and minerals in the body. The micronutrients are required in small quantities, and they are essential in doing everything from regulating hormones to boosting brain performance. Macros are also different from the macrobiotic diet, which has principles drawn from Zen Buddhism.

## Keto Diet Macros Between Men and Women After 50

Macros zero in on the composition of your daily calories so that you can alter each to give you the best health that you want. If you have 70% calories in carbs, then you will feel different, unlike when you have 70% calories from fats. Men and women after 50 have to understand their macros so that they can adjust them according to their health and energy needs. With tracking, you can understand the source of the imbalance and make changes that will promote better growth and development of new cells. Many people on a ketogenic diet will make the mistake of counting calories alone. This will not give them meaningful results because you will not know the balance of your energy source. If you want a more productive approach, you should monitor your macronutrients because it will tell you a more decent and better approach that you can use to achieve your health goals. Besides, when you follow the quality of your macros, you can potentially increase your fat-burning abilities and have a lean body.

## Counting macros

Keto macros are everything. Simply put, your body needs a certain ratio of macronutrients (carbohydrates, fats, and proteins) to maintain ketosis.

Carbohydrates should make up less than 5% of your calorie intake. At the beginning of the diet, it is recommended to consume less than 20 g per day. A good ratio is 1.5 grams of net carbs per 100 calories.

When following a ketogenic diet, you should keep track of your net carbs. This calculation is pretty simple: Net Carbs = Total Carbohydrates - Fiber.

For example, one cup (91 grams) of broccoli contains 6 grams of carbs and 2.4 grams of fiber. This means that one cup of broccoli contains 3.6 grams of carbohydrates. We count net carbs because dietary fiber has no significant metabolic effect, which means it doesn't raise blood sugar.

When carbohydrates are removed from the diet, it is easy to replace them with protein, but eating foods high in protein does not promote ketosis. To properly switch your body to use fat for fuel, your protein content must be moderate.

A moderate amount of protein is 1.2-1.7 g of protein per day per 1 kg of body weight. That is, if you weigh 70 kg, then you need to consume about 85-110 g of protein per day.

Now let's talk about fat. Fat is what makes you complete, energizes (in ketosis) and makes food tasty. For most people, this figure should be 70% of the daily calories. Keep carbs under 20g, eat moderate amounts of protein, and eat fat until you're full

At first, you may overeat calories, but over time, the keto diet will automatically fix this. Your diet and natural hunger signals will automatically adjust.

Here's a quick example of the daily breakdown of macronutrients on a keto diet at about 2,000 calories per day:

• 80 calories / 20 grams net carbs

• 320 calories / 80 grams protein

• 1200 calories / 133 grams of fat

Again, the total calories you eat isn't as important as controlling your macros. For an accurate calculation, use our keto calculator.

## Calculating Your Daily Caloric Intake

Many people are of the opinion that calculating your calories while you are on keto diet is not very important, but it is always good to keep a watch on how many calories you are consuming a day. You should calculate how much calories you get to consume every day by having an idea of how much weight you want to lose.

If your body needs 2,000 calories a day but you consume only 1400 then your body is in a caloric deficit so it will have to tap into the fat reserves of your body. This will result in loss of weight. There are various calculators available online which can be used to calculate your daily caloric intake considering your objectives, age, height, activity level along with other factors.

In general, if you want to lose weight, you need to subtract around 600 calories from your daily caloric needs. So less than 1,000-1,200 calories if you are a woman and less than 1400-1600 calories if you are a man.

## The Calorie and Nutrient Balance

Do you know why else the Ketogenic Diet is good for you specifically, as someone who just hit 50 years of age? What you should keep in mind is that as a person advances in age, their calorie needs decrease. For example, instead of 2,000 calories per day – you'll need only 1,800 calories per day. Why is that? Well, when we start to age –our physical activity significantly decreases. Hence, we don't need as much energy in our system. However, that doesn't mean our nutrient needs also go down. We still need the same number of vitamins and minerals.

The Ketogenic Diet manages to hit a balance between these two needs. You get high nutrition for every calorie you get – which means that you'll maintain a decent amount of weight without really feeling less energetic for day to day activities.

## Having a Meal Plan

When you have a complete meal, plan laid out in front of you, you are in a better position to have an idea as to what your diet would look like in the days to come. If you have to spontaneously decide what you are going to prepare to eat every time you are in the kitchen, chances of you getting off the rails become pretty high.

You can start off by first calculating how much calories a day you are going to consume.

The next step would be to decide which macronutrients will have to be incorporated and in what proportion in order for your body to reach that goal. Remember that the rule of thumb is 75:20:5 for Fats: Proteins: Carbs, respectively.

## Finding Out Good Recipes

If you eat the same boring food every day you won't be able to sustain on this diet for a long time and you might get distracted pretty soon. Try to find a good variety of recipes. Maybe you can eat some eggs in the morning and tuna at night or maybe a good wholesome salad one time and a full fat yogurt the other time that will keep your boat afloat.

When it comes to meal plans, it is very subjective so go with whatever you feel comfortable with but make sure to keep these guiding principles in sight:

1. Do not go about eating same food all the time. Monotony will bore you very soon.

2. Stick with the "concept of keto" by consuming as low carbs as you can.

3. Fats and proteins should come from healthy sources most of the time.

4. A low carb fried chicken or some other fried product here and there will not hurt much but it should be kept at a bare minimum level.

## What is Ketosis?

Ketosis is a metabolic state where the body is efficiently using fat for energy. In a regular diet, carbohydrates produce glucose, which is used to provide energy. Glucose is stored in the body in fat cells that travel via the bloodstream. People gain weight when there is fatter stored than being used as energy.

Glucose is formed through the consumption of sugar and starch. Namely carbohydrates. The sugars may be in the form of natural sugars from fruit or milk, or they may be formed from processed sugar. Starches like pasta, rice or starchy vegetables like potatoes and corn, form glucose as well. The body breaks down the sugars from these foods into glucose. Glucose and insulin combined to help carry glucose into the bloodstream so the body can use glucose as energy. The glucose that is not used is stored in the liver and muscles.

In order for the body to supply ketones for use as fuel, the body must use up all the reserves of glucose. In order to do this, there must be a condition of the body of starvation low carbohydrates, passing, or strenuous exercise. An exceptionally low carb diet, the production of ketones what her to feel the body and brain.

Ketones are produced from the liver when there is not enough glucose in the body to provide energy. When insulin levels are low, and there is not enough glucose or sugar in the bloodstream, fat is released from fat cells and travels in the blood to the liver. The liver processes the fat into ketones. Ketones are released into the bloodstream to provide fuel for the body and increase the body's metabolism. Ketones are formed under conditions of starvation, fasting, or a diet low in carbohydrates.

## How to Enter Ketosis?

You have a few options when it comes to entering ketosis. The most direct one is by depriving your body of carbohydrates, therefore glucose, through fasting for a long period. When you stop eating altogether, your body will turn to burn fat as a source of energy because it has no glucose to work with.

# Disadvantages

Your body will have an adjustment period. It depends from person to person on how many days that will be, but when you start any new diet or exercise routine, your body has to adjust to the new normal. With the keto diet, you are drastically cutting your carbohydrates intake, so the body has to adjust to that. You may feel slow, weak, fatigued, and like you are not thinking as quick or fast as you used to. It just means your body is adjusting to keto and once this adjustment period is done, you will see the weight loss results you anticipated.

If you are an athlete, you may need more carbohydrates. If you still want to try keto as an athlete, it's important you talk to your nutritionist or trainer to see how the diet can be tweaked for you. Most athletes require a greater intake of carbs than the keto diet requires which means they may have to up their intake in order to assure they have the energy for their training sessions. High endurance sports (like rugby or soccer) and heavy weightlifting do require a greater intake of carbohydrates. If you're an athlete wanting to follow keto and gain the health benefits, it's important you first talk to your trainer before making any changes to your diet.

You have to carefully count your daily macros! For beginners, this can be tough, and even people already on keto can become lazy about this. People are often used to eating what they want without worrying about just how many grams of protein or carbs it contains. With keto, you have to be meticulous about counting your intake to ensure you are maintaining the necessary keto breakdown (75% fat, 20% protein, ~5% carbs). The closer you stick to this, the better results you will see regarding weight loss and other health benefits. If your weight loss has stalled or you're not feeling as energetic as you hoped, it could be because your macros are off. Find a free calorie counting app that and be sure you look at the ingredients of everything you're eating and cooking.

# CHAPTER 2:

# How to Get Started with the Ketogenic Diet When You're Over 50?

## How Aging Affects Your Nutritional Needs?

Nutrition is vital in maintaining a healthy biological system. You can lead a happy and fulfilling life when you choose the right nutrition. However, it is imperative to understand that nutrition changes with age, and if you are suffering from nutritional deficiencies, then it will bring harmful outcomes. In the initial years of childhood, the little bodies will require essential nutrients to enable them to grow and develop quickly, both physically and mentally. The food should provide high energy as well as nourishing abilities that can enhance the cognitive abilities of the child. It is also important to note that the child is learning new foods and developing their taste, which will shape their eating habits in the future.

Therefore, the kids should be encouraged to consume a wide array of foods to help them get all the essential nutrients. The key nutrient includes proteins which are necessary for growth, Vitamin D to help in the growth of strong bones. Along with other vital nutrients such as vitamin A is vital in boosting the immune system, while zinc and iron are essential in boosting the mental abilities of the kids.

# How to Start a Keto Diet When You are Over 50?

## Consult a Nutrition Specialist

This book is a valuable tool to get an idea of what a ketogenic diet is, what the benefits are, and how to avoid the classic mistakes. It is a complete guide, with which, if studied well, you will certainly be able to set your diet according to your daily needs. However, consulting a doctor is never a bad idea; you can discuss your opinions and can give you valuable advice. I recommend consulting your doctor especially in cases of health problems and in cases where you have never been on a diet.

## Don't Forget to Eat Starchy Vegetables

Don't overdo it with proteins. Remember that we are always talking about a diet, so you will still have a certain calorie deficit. This is always true, but it is especially true for the ketogenic diet. Taking the right dose of protein is fine, taking a little more is not a problem, but taking a lot more, yes. It is for two reasons, the first and most important is that the body has a certain ability to assimilate proteins, if this is greatly exceeded, some organs, including the liver, may not function well. Second reason, if you do not create an energy deficit, you will never lose weight.

## Drink and Consume Electrolytes (water, herbal teas, fresh juices)

Do you remember the previous point when I said, "taking on a little more isn't a problem"? Perfect, to be even more precise: taking a little more is not a problem if taking the right amount of liquids. You can't do it differently, we should always drink a lot, but this is even more true in cases where we decide to follow a ketogenic diet: liquids are used by the organs to dispose of all proteins, if we don't drink, if we don't dilute proteins , the organs will suffer and we will have many other problems.

# Keto Diet and Aging

Keto nourishments convey a high measure of sustenance per calorie. This is significant because basal metabolic rate (the measure of calories required every day to endure) is less for seniors, however, despite everything, they need an indistinguishable measure of supplements from more youthful individuals.

An individual aged 50+ will have a lot harder time living on low-quality nourishments than a high schooler or 20-something whose body is flexible.

This makes it significantly increasingly urgent for seniors to eat nourishments that are wellbeing supporting and ailment battling. It can truly mean the contrast between getting a charge out of the brilliant years without limit or spending them in torment and distress.

In this manner, seniors need to eat a progressively ideal eating routine by keeping away from "void calories "from sugars or nourishments wealthy in enemies of supplements, for example, entire grains, and expanding their measure of supplement rich fats and proteins.

It is critical to monitor Ketogenic Diet by following your solid eating regimen with an exceptional clinical instrument at home without consulting your primary care physician each time.

Keto diets offer plenty of vitamins per calorie. This is vital because you are older; you need fewer calories. However, you still need an identical amount of vitamins as you did in your younger days. You could have a stricter time residing on junk food, not like when you had been younger. This approach is essential to eat foods that guide your health and fight diseases. This can help you live an exciting lifestyle while getting old gracefully. You want to take in more magnificent optimal meals and avoid immoderate and empty calories observed in sugar-wealthy foods like grains. You want to increase the amount of nutrient-wealthy proteins and fat you consume.

Carb-rich ingredients are pushed using society and aren't beneficial to your long term health. Carb low diets containing excessive quantities of plant and animal fat are way better for increasing insulin sensitivity. It also slows down cognitive decline, making your overall health higher.

It's never too late to enhance your possibilities of functioning and feeling as you get older. You can start doing better by eating better. Keto for girls over 50 years is another danger to repair some of the damage performed in your younger days while you didn't pay attention to what you ate.

The more in advance you begin to make those changes to enhance your weight, immunity, and blood sugar, the better your chances of living better and longer.

In conclusion, all of us get older. However, we will all control our satisfaction with life as we get even older. Keto diets assist you in enhancing your health so that you can thrive instead of being in pains and illness as you get farther away from fifty.

# Why it is Hard to Lose Weight After 50?

As a woman, you have likely experienced significant differences in the way that you must diet compared to the way that men can diet. Women tend to have a harder time losing weight because of their different hormones and the way their bodies break down fats. Another factor to consider is your age group. As the body ages, it is important to be more attentive with the way that you care for yourself. Aging bodies start to experience problems more quickly and this can be avoided with the proper diet and exercise plan. Keto works well for women of all ages and this is because of how it communicates with the body. No matter how fit you are right now or how much weight you need or want to lose, Keto is going to change the way that your body metabolizes, giving you a very personalized experience.

When starting your Keto diet, you should not be thinking about extremes because that isn't what Keto should be about. You should be able to place your body into ketosis without feeling terrible in the process. One of the biggest guidelines to follow while starting your Keto journey is that you need to listen to your body regularly. If you ever feel that you are starving or simply unfulfilled, then you will likely have to modify the way you are eating because it isn't reaching ketosis properly. It is not an overnight journey, so you need to remember to be patient with yourself and with your body. Adapting to a Keto diet takes a bit of transition time and a lot of awareness.

Your metabolism is unique, but it is also going to be slower than a man's by nature. Since muscle is able to burn more calories than fat, the weight just seems to fall off of men, giving them the ability to reach the opportunity for muscle growth quickly. This should not be something that holds you back from starting your Keto journey. As long as you are keeping these realistic bodily factors in mind, you won't be left wondering why it is taking you a little bit longer to start losing weight. This point will come for you, but it will take a little bit more of a process that you must be committed to following through with.

When the body begins to successfully run on fats, you have an automatic fuel reserve waiting to be burned. It will take some time for your body to do this, but when it does, you will actually be able to eat fewer calories and still feel just as full because your body knows to take energy from the fat that you already have. This will become automatic. It is, however, a process that requires some patience, but being aware of what is actually going on with your body can help you stay motivated while on Keto.

Because a Keto diet reduces the amount of sugar you are consuming, it naturally lowers the amount of insulin in your bloodstream. This can actually have amazing effects on any existing PCOS and fertility issues, as well as menopausal symptoms and conditions like prediabetes and Type 2 diabetes. Once your body adjusts to a Keto diet, you are overcoming the things that are naturally in place that can be preventing you from losing weight and getting healthy. Even if you placed your body on a strict diet, if it isn't getting rid of sugars properly, you likely aren't going to see the same results that you will when you try Keto. This is a big reason why Keto can be so beneficial for women.

# CHAPTER 3:

# Keto Diet for Seniors

## Keto Diet for Women Over 50

Women who are looking for a quick and effective way to shed excess weight, get high blood sugar levels under control, reduce overall inflammations, and improve physical and mental energy will do their best by following a ketogenic diet plan. But there are special considerations women must take into account when they are beginning the keto diet.

All women know it is much more difficult for women to lose weight than it is for men to lose weight. A woman will live on a starvation level diet, exercise like a triathlete, and only lose five pounds. A man will stop putting dressing on his salad and will lose twenty pounds. It just is not fair. But we have the fact that we are women to blame. Women naturally have more standing between them and weight loss than men do.

The mere fact that we are women is the single largest contributor to the reason we find it difficult to lose weight. Since our bodies always think they need to be prepared for the possibility of pregnancy women will naturally have more body fat and less mass in our muscles than men will. Muscle cells burn more calories than fat cells do. So, because we are women, we will always lose weight more slowly than men will.

Being in menopause will also cause women to add more pounds to their bodies, especially in the lower half of the body. After menopause a woman's metabolism naturally slows down. Your hormones levels will decrease. These two factors alone will cause weight gain in the post-menopausal woman.

Women are a direct product of their hormones. Men also have hormones but not the ones like we have that regulate every function in our bodies. And the hormones in women will fluctuate around their everyday habits like lack of sleep, poor eating habits, and menstrual cycles. These hormones cause women to crave sweets around the time their periods occur. These cravings will wreck any diet plan. Staying true to the keto plan is challenging at this time because of the intense craving for sweets and carbs. Also having your period will often make you feel and look bloated because of the water your body holds onto during this time. And having cramps make you more likely to reach for a bag of cookies than a plate of steak and salad.

Because we are women, we may experience challenges on the keto diet that men will not face because they are men. One of these challenges is having weight loss plateau or even experiencing weight gain. This can happen because of the influence of hormones on weight loss in women. If this happens you will want to increase your consumption of good fats like ghee, butter, eggs, coconut oil, beef, avocados, and olive oil. Any food that is cooked or prepared using oil must be prepared in olive oil or avocado oil.

You can also use MCT oil. MCT stands for Medium Chain Triglycerides. This is a form of fatty acid that is saturated and has many health benefits. MCT can help with many body functions from weight loss to improved brain function. MCTs are mostly missing from the typical American diet because we have been told that saturated fats are harmful to the body, and as a group they are. But certain saturated fats, like MCTs, are actually beneficial to the body, especially when they come from good foods like beef or coconut oil. They are easier to digest than most other saturated fats and may help improve heart and brain function and prevent obesity.

Many women on a keto diet will struggle with imbalances in their hormones. On the keto diet you do not rely on lowered calories to lose weight but on foods effect on your hormones. So, when women begin the keto diet any issues, they are already having with their hormones will be brought to attention and may cause the woman to give up before she really begins. Always remember that the keto diet is responsible for cleansing the system first so that the body can easily respond to the wonderful affects a keto diet has to offer.

Do not try to work toward the lean body that many men sport. It is best for overall function that women stay at twenty-two to twenty-six percent body fat. Our hormones will function best in this range and we can't possibly function without our hormones. Women who are very lean, like gymnasts and extreme athletes, will find their hormones no longer function or function at a less than optimal rate. And remember that ideal weight may not be the right weight for you. Many women find that they perform their best when they are at their happy weight. If you find yourself fighting with yourself to lose the last few pounds you think you need to lose in order to have the perfect body, then it may not be worth it. The struggle will affect your hormone function. Carefully observing the keto diet will allow time for your hormones to stabilize and regulate themselves back to their pre-obesity normal function.

Like any other diet plan the keto diet will work better if you are active. Regular exercise will allow the body to strengthen and tone muscles and will help to work off excess fat reserves. But exercise requires energy to accomplish. If you restrict your carb intake too much you might not have the energy needed to be physically able to make it all the way through the day and still be able to maintain an exercise routine. You might need to add in more carbs to your diet through the practice of carb cycling.

As a woman you know that sometimes your emotions get the better of you. This is true with your body, as you well know, and can be a major reason why women find it extremely difficult at times to lose weight the way they want to lose weight. We have been led to believe that not only can we do it all but that we must do it all. This gives many women unnecessary levels of pressure and can cause them to engage in emotional eating. Some women might have lowered feelings of self-worth and may not feel they are entitled to the benefits of the keto diet and turning to food relieves the feelings of inadequacy that we try to hide from the world.

When you engage in the same activity for a long period of time it becomes a habit. When you reach for the bag of potato chips or the tub of ice cream whenever you are angry, upset, or depressed, then your brain will eventually tell you to reach for food whenever you feel an emotion that you don't want to deal with. Food acts as a security blanket against the world outside. It may be necessary to address any extreme emotional issues you are having before you begin the keto diet, so that you are better assured of success.

The basic act of staying on the keto diet can be incredibly challenging for some women. Many women see beginning a new diet to lose weight as a punishment for being overweight. It may be worthwhile for you to work at changing the set of your mind if you are feeling this way. You may need to remind yourself daily that the keto diet is not a punishment but a blessing for your body. Tell yourself that you are not denying yourself certain foods because you can't eat them, but because you do not like the way those foods make your body feel. Don't watch other people eating their high carb diet and pity yourself. Instead, feel sorry for the people who have trapped themselves in a high calorie diet and are not experiencing the benefits that you are experiencing.

For the first thirty days cut out all sweeteners, even the non-sugar ones that are allowed on the keto diet. While they may make food taste better, they also remind your brain that it needs sweet foods when it really doesn't. Cutting them out for at least thirty days will break the cycle that your body has fallen into and will cut the cravings for sweets in your diet.

It is very possible for women to be successful on the keto diet if they are prepared to follow a few simple adjustments that will make the diet look differently than your male partner might be eating but that will make you successful in the long run.

During the first one or two weeks you will need to consume extra fat than a man might need to. Doing this will have three important effects on your body. First it will cause your mitochondria to intensify their acceptance of your new way of finding energy. Mitochondria are tiny organisms that are found in cells and are responsible for using the fuel that insulin brings to the cell for fuel for the cell. Increasing your fat intake will also help make sure you are getting enough calories in your daily diet. This is important because if your body thinks you are starving, it will begin to conserve calories and you will stop losing weight.

The third benefit from eating more fat, and perhaps the most important, is the psychological boost you will get from seeing that you can eat more fat and still lose weight and feel good. It will also reset your mindset that you formerly might have held against fat. For so long we have been told that low fat is the only way to lose weight. But an absence of dietary fat will lead to overeating and binge eating out of a feeling of deprivation. When you begin the diet by allowing yourself to eat a lot, or too much in your mind, fat, then you swing the pendulum around to the other side of the fat scale where it properly belongs. You teach yourself that fat

29 | P a g .

can be good for you. Increasing the extra intake of fats should not last beyond the second week of the diet. Your body will improve its abilities to create and burn ketones and body fat, and then you will begin using your own body fat for fuel and you can begin to lower your reliance on dietary fat a little bit so that you will begin to lose weight.

The keto diet is naturally lower in calories if you follow the recommended levels of food intake. It is not necessary to try to restrict your intake of calories even further. All you need to do is to eat only until you are full and not one bite more. Besides losing weight, the aim of the keto diet is to retrain your body on how to work properly. You will need to learn to trust your body and the signals it sends out to be able to readjust to a proper way of eating.

## Menopause

There comes an age in a woman's life where her menstrual cycle will finally end. This is a phase that means your ovaries stop releasing eggs, better known as ovulation, and therefore menstruation ends. This condition is generally observed in women above the age of 40. There is no defined age that shows when a woman can expect menopause.

There are times where women may experience menopause prematurely as well. This happens if a woman has undergone surgeries like hysterectomy (surgery that involves removal of ovaries). It can also happen from any injuries that may have caused damage to the ovaries. If this happens before the age of 40, it is classified as premature menopause.

Menopause, as harmless as it sounds, can be quite a troubling phase for women. The hot flashes you experience will keep you up at night, with an elevated heartbeat. The constant feeling of being irritated and a clear downfall in your sex life can contribute greatly towards you feeling more and more grumpy.

Menopause takes a toll on your hormonal balance and the newly developed imbalance then pushes your body to gain massive weight, experience mood swings like never before and a libido that is crashing faster than you can imagine.

If you think this is bad, here are some other issues that menopause can lead to:

- Chronic stress

- Anxiety

- Insulin spike

- Type 2 Diabetes

- Heart Diseases

- Polycystic Ovary Syndrome (PCOS)

The overall picture, then, is grim! Fortunately, a difference of lifestyle and a carefully thought-out diet plan can change all that for you. I am not saying it happens overnight or within a week, but the profound impacts are felt rather quick. In the longer run, keto will rescue you and your body from impending doom and allow you to lead a life without worrying about keeping a glucose monitor or any of the typical health-related equipment near you.

The keto diet, while there are many classes of it, helps your hormones to remain in shape and balanced. This means that you do not have to worry about the insulin or any other hormones, hence minimizing the hot flashes and other symptoms. Even if they occur, they will be minor and far less painful.

Moreover, the keto diet jump-starts your sex drive. The fat-rich diet improves fat-soluble vitamin absorption. Not to forget it especially helps with vitamin D, a vital piece that goes missing with age. All in all, this provides all the drive you need to have intimate moments even in your fifties.

## **Heart Diseases**

Keto diets help women over 50 to shed those extra pounds. Reducing any amount of weight greatly reduces the chances of a heart attack or any other heart complications. Through the carefully selected diet routine, not only are you losing weight and enjoying scrumptious meals, but you are significantly boosting your heart's health and reviving yourself from the otherwise dull state that you may have been in before.

## Diabetes Control

Needless to say, the careful selection of ingredients, when cooked together, provide rich nutrients, free from any processed or harmful contents such as sugar. Add to that the fact that keto automatically controls your insulin levels. The result is a glucose level that is always under control and continued control would lead to a day where you will say goodbye to the medications you might be taking for diabetes. And so Much More!

By taking up the challenge and adapting the keto way, you are ensuring yourself one of the safest journeys into the older years, if not the safest of the lot. Sure, there will be days where you may miss a food or two, but that craving will be overshadowed by the benefits the keto diet will bring for you.

With the help of the keto diet, you can expect a few more benefits such as:

- Improved and stable blood pressure levels

- A deeper sleep for those suffering from insomnia

- Improved kidney function

- More energy that lasts all day

- Improved bodily functions All Set to Begin?

Great! Let me be the first one to let you know that you are not too late to start. The fact is, no one is ever too late to change their eating, sleeping, and working habits. All it takes is a spark of motivation, and if you are reading this line, you already have that spark. All you need now is to grab a pen and a paper to note down some fine recipes and jot down the things you need and the things you should avoid. Better yet, maintain a little diary or a notebook which you can refer to whenever you wish.

## Balance Hormones

As we all know, menopause causes a major hormonal imbalance, keto has been proven to help create a balance in hormones including estrogen. By creating a balance in hormones, it helps to control hot flashes that most women experience after menopause. Not only do older women benefit by this, but keto can help treat premenstrual symptoms in younger women too.

## Enhances Brain Function

Estrogen helps in ensuring that glucose can seamlessly flow into the brain. As the estrogen levels begin to lower after menopause, the glucose levels reaching the brain also decrease. This can drastically lower the function of your brain. However, keto helps to maintain a smooth flow of glucose in the brain, which enhances the brain functions.

# Keto Diet for Men Over 50

Men much like women, also go through quite a lot of internal and external changes. These include but are not limited to physical changes, habitual changes, and so on. While the chemistry inside the body of both remains broadly the same, whether young or old, there are things which men are more likely to develop or lose than women. These include some diseases, ailments, infections, habitual changes, and disorders. The worst news is, it happens as soon as you cross 45 years of age. That means you are at least five years late already, or at least that is what you think.

However, unlike most diets which you can begin right away, there are a few things I should point out which men should keep an eye out for. Consider these as soft reminders or suggestions before you take up the keto challenge.

## Keto Diet is a Lifestyle

It is not a diet that you do for a few weeks and then resume your normal food and carb intake. This is a proper lifestyle that you will need to adopt and live with. As long as you continue abiding by its rules, you will continue to enjoy the benefits it has to offer.

## Keto is not Only Meant for Women

There are those who actually believe that keto was designed specifically for women. I am here to set things right and let you know that keto is for both men and women.

## Keto Does not Require You to Cut Down on Your Eating Habits

Not at all. With that said though, it does make you modify those habits by changing what you consume instead of how much you consume.

## Keto Food Items May Pose a Risk to People with Special Medical Conditions

It is something that most websites, blogs, and articles fail to mention. If you suffer from issues like high cholesterol, be sure to do a bit of research regarding what you can use instead of a specific ingredient.

With that said, let us get down to details and find out just why keto is so important for men who are 50 years old and above.

50 Marks the Start of Troubles Well, in all fairness, troubles for men may start a little sooner than that, but the reason I said that is because some of these troubles, such as diseases or issues related to obesity and weight gain, take some time to manifest themselves. It is usually around the 50-year mark where these issues come up almost immediately.

Now that you are within this age group, and are nearing your retirement age, there are so many things which can cause you to lose your patience, your focus, and depreciate your health as well. The biggest of these would be stress; the stress of not knowing what you will do once you have retired.

This stress can cause you to have insomnia, a massive eating disorder, and ultimately a body that is quickly running out of shape. With each passing year, you are incurring extra expenses upon yourself and trying to find shirt and trousers that fits your new size. I completely understand that none of us, men, or women, like to see that.

Stress is just the start of things; I haven't even begun to point out the medical issues a man's body can develop and be bombarded with. To give you an idea of what a 50-year-old male faces who is not observing any kind of diet, here is a list to digest:

- Anxiety

- Depression

- Uncontrollable blood pressure levels

- Diminishing sex drive

- Increased laziness

- Lack of energy

Fluctuating insulin levels Think about it, do any of these really sound the sort of issues you would be okay to face in such an age? Certainly, you need some form of assistance that can help you boost your morale, your spirits, and allow you to control life the way you had always done so.

"Exercise is the answer!" Well, yes and no.

You see, while exercise provides you with the muscular strength and some really good benefits, it is still not the ideal way to cut down on those extra pounds, nor will it allow you to control other bodily disorders. All exercise can do is to keep your body in shape physically. That is all there is to it. There is a simple reason for that.

Exercises are designed to utilize your body's energy and use it to carry out difficult tasks which, as a result, promote more strength and growth of muscles and mass. The keyword to focus here is "energy" and that is exactly where a diet comes in. In this case, we will be focusing on possibly the best diet of them all: keto.

The good news is that by combining your love of keto and exercise, you end up with the perfect duo that is always ready to complement each other. While they do that, you, the actual end-user, gets to enjoy a perfectly healthy lifestyle that is free from any harmful carbs or other nutrients.

For men over the age of 50, it is very much important to remain in good shape. This is something you would want to do as it allows you to carry out more tasks relatively easy and keeps you active throughout the day. But wait, there is more to keto than just that.

## Helping You Live Longer

Through adopting a keto diet plan for your meals, and adding exercise to that, you are most likely to lead a longer life. Why do I say this? If you haven't noticed already, the keto diet comes with quite a lot of benefits.

The keto diet helps you to improve your blood sugar levels. This eliminates quite a lot of issues such as type 2 diabetes. Additionally, the keto plan helps you in keeping carbs at bay. This in return pushes your body to absorb fats as fuel instead. By doing so, your body will start to burn fats quicker than usual, and that is some good news for everyone.

As you grow old, some functions fade out while others slow down to a snail's pace. An example of the latter is the rate at which our body burns fat now versus how it used to burn fat when you were younger. There is a significant difference, and with keto you can recover that ability fairly easy as it trains your body to switch into ketosis mode.

This new change within your body would then make room for more energy. The more energy you have, the better you can work, focus, and carry out tasks. Finally, the keto diet never asks you to stop eating, and that means you always have a healthy meal waiting for you at least three times a day, if not more.

Combine all that and your body automatically starts to feel fresher and healthier. This will also have a drastic effect on your personality. With more confidence, you will be able to deal with the public and lead a happier life.

## Boosts Testosterone Levels

Lower testosterone levels are highly associated with increased body fat, insomnia, and loss of muscle mass. As mentioned above, keto does an excellent job in boosting testosterone level, meaning you'll have yourself feeling more energized than before.

## Improves Sexual Drive

As men grow older, low sex drive and testosterone levels can be a problem. This can often lead to decreased energy level and even loss of muscle mass. To counter this, consuming high levels of fat has actually been known to increase testosterone levels by 13%. This also works well to reduce irritability and mood imbalance which is of course a win-win!

Keto diets have been known to have significant impact on the composition of hormones. For more questions, you can reach out to a professional.

## Good Under the Sheets

Let's be honest, we all have a few things on our priority list which we cannot compromise on. One of them is sharing those intimate moments with our partner, right? The bad part is the libido, the thing that makes this magic possible, starts to drop low as we approach the half-century mark. Once we cross that, the fall increases drastically, and we feel the lack of urge for intimacy and a lower sex drive.

When something as important and pleasurable as sex dies out, life takes a toll. Without it, both men and women grow grumpy, irritated and lose their charm. While women have to worry about the menopause issues, men get to deal with things like erectile dysfunction. In either case, it is the stuff of nightmares.

With the help of keto though, things can change and change for the better. With a selection of some fine ingredients, you can cook up some food that will top your body up with the energy, strength, and the libido that you need to get back in action. Add to that a few exercises, and you would be as fit as you were quite a few years younger. Relive the moments with your loved ones and rekindle the fire that seemingly went out for good.

## Strengthening the Bones

One of the biggest issues' men face when they cross the magical number of 50 is the rapidly deteriorating strength within their bones. While they may have been able to walk for miles without breaking a sweat, back in the day, they would now face an incredibly tough time climbing a set of stairs no more than two stories high. This is an alarming situation, and one that needs a solution ASAP!

Fortunately, the keto diet provides some relief to the people suffering from joint aches from osteoarthritis and weakened muscles. Through this diet, the necessary nutrients are released into the body which will then cause a sudden spike within the body, brimming it with energy to carry out tasks that would otherwise seem impossible to do at such an age.

Imagine the keto diet as spinach for Popeye. The minute he eats it, he's all muscles. I should also point out that this is just a reference and that keto does not provide you with such quick results.

## Keto Helps to Prevent Certain Cancers

Cancer, whatever the type, is one of the most horrific diseases in existence. Just the mere mention of the word and everyone will immediately be stunned.

Cancers take time to manifest and are usually caused by long prevailing, underlying causes. They do not appear randomly and require the right kind of environment to develop. However, once they appear, time is of the essence. Be late and it is curtains for good.

With the introduction of keto, which was initially introduced within children to control epilepsy, things looked promising. While keto does not prevent all cancers, it is mighty effective against some types of cancers. Some reports have shown significant revival of patients who were aged 50 and above, which provides all the more reason for men above 50 to start on ketogenic diets, if they haven't already done so. Simply put, keto is possibly the only lifestyle men should seek to ensure a healthier life leading into retirement.

## Some Side Affects You Should Know

Some of these side effects are universal, meaning that both men and women would face these. However, there are varying studies which suggest some symptoms or side-effects are more prominent within men above 50 as compared to women above 50. Nonetheless, it is a good idea to know what exactly you are dealing with and what you can expect to face as time goes by.

Most of these symptoms will fade away with time, but some may linger on. There is no such symptom that may pose a threat to you or anyone else. However, it is generally a good idea to be prepared to face these as they come. A prepared mind stands a better chance at dealing with things.

The side-effects, if you haven't already read the women's section, include:

## 1.     The Dreaded Keto Flu

A flu like illness that hits you right in the starting few weeks. Nothing to be alarmed about as this is only because your body is coping with the new changes.

## 2.     Keto Breath

I do wish this was not the case, but since it exists, it is best to know of it beforehand. Keto breath is quite strong as it contains acetone.

## 3.     Tougher Visits to the Bathroom

You can either develop diarrhea or nasty constipation. However, rest assured, this is a short-term symptom and will go away shortly.

## 4.     A Massive Thirst

Yes! You will feel thirsty quite a lot. It is advisable that you drink plenty of water to ensure you do not suffer worse side-effects because of the added thirst.

Some of these symptoms may be more noticeable for men than women. However, the difference is marginal at best.

You will be spending a lot of time in the kitchen, so it is probably a good idea to hone in on your cooking skills. You will need them quite a lot if you truly wish to take benefits from the keto diet.

# Benefits of Keto for Seniors After 50

There are a lot of benefits in starting a ketogenic diet, be it in terms of weight, experience or to improve your health!

## Effective in Fighting Epilepsy

The primary goal of this diet, introduced in Antiquity, was to fight against epilepsy. The ketones may affect anti-convulsion, but to date it is not possible to say why they have this effect on the body.

## Effective in Weight Loss

Your body's source of energy in the ketogenic diet is fat, either from food or stored by your body. This therefore has advantages: the level of insulin, a hormone that stores fat, drops very significantly, this means that your body will become more efficient at burning fat.

## Cholesterol and Blood Pressure

Diabetes and high blood pressure are some of the most common reasons that result in death among older adults. Keto diet is effective in this regard because it improves triglyceride and cholesterol levels that are associated with arterial buildups. It also leads to an increase in high-density lipoprotein (HDL) and decreases in low-density lipoprotein (LDL) particles. All of this comes together to the improvement in blood pressure.

## Regulate Blood Sugar

Keto diet helps regulate blood sugar by controlling how much insulin is in the system. Maintaining the right level of insulin is important because you can avoid problems such as insulin resistance or pre-diabetes. Keto diet has also been shown to reduce HbA1c levels, which is a measure of blood glucose control.

## Fights Neurological Disorders

Keto diet has been used in the past to treat neurological disorders or other cognitive impairments such as epilepsy. When your body goes into ketosis, your body produces ketones that help reverse neurodegenerative illnesses. Here, the brain just uses another source of energy instead of using the cellular energy pathway that is faulty in people with brain disorders. That means the keto diet can help prevent or treat disorders such as Parkinson's and Alzheimer's.

## Helps You Lose Weight

For most people, this is the first and foremost benefit of switching to keto! Their former diet method may have stalled for them or they were starting to notice weight creeping back on. With keto, studies have shown that people have been able to follow this diet and relay fewer hunger pangs and suppressed appetite while losing weight at the same time!

## Improve Cardiovascular Risk Symptoms to Overall Lower Your Chances of Having Heart Disease

Most people assume that following keto that is so high in fat content has to increase your risk of coronary heart disease or heart attack. But the research proves otherwise! Research shows that switching to keto can lower your blood pressure, increase your HDL good cholesterol, and reduce your triglyceride fatty acid levels. That's because the fats you are consuming on keto are healthy and high-quality fats, so they tend to reverse many unhealthy symptoms of heart disease.

## Increases the Body's Energy Levels

We briefly compared the difference between the glucose molecules synthesized from a high carbohydrates intake versus ketones produced on the keto diet. Ketones are made by the liver and use fat molecules you already have stored. This makes them much more energy-rich and a lasting source of fuel compared to glucose, a simple sugar molecule. These ketones can give you a burst of energy physically as well as mentally allow you to have greater focus, clarity, and attention to detail.

## Decreases Inflammation in the Body

Inflammation on its own is a natural response by the body's immune system, but when it becomes uncontrollable, it can lead to an array of health problems, some severe, some minor. The many health concerns include acne, autoimmune conditions, arthritis, psoriasis, irritable bowel syndrome, and even acne and eczema.

## Increases Your Mental Functioning Level

Like we elaborated earlier, the energy-rich ketones can boost the body's physical and mental levels of alertness. Research has shown that keto is a much better energy source for the brain than simple sugar glucose molecules are. With nearly 75% of your diet coming from healthy fats, the brain's neural cells and mitochondria have a better source of energy to be able to function at the highest level.

## Can Regulate Hormones in Women Who Have Pcos And Pms

Women who have PCOS (polycystic ovary syndrome) suffer from infertility which can be very heartbreaking for young couples trying to start a family. There is no cure for this condition, but it is believed that it is related to many similar diabetic symptoms like obesity and high insulin levels. This causes the body to produce more sex hormones which can lead to infertility. The keto diet has become a popular method to try and regulate insulin and hormone levels and could increase a woman's chances of getting pregnant.

## Effective in People with Alzheimer's

The ketogenic diet is effective in the treatment of neurodegenerative diseases like Alzheimer because it aims to increase the enzymes of the mitochondrial metabolism. Clearly, this would develop more energy in the brain, and therefore improve cognitive efficiency.

In addition to all this, the ketogenic diet would have a role in protecting against oxidative stress, and therefore would be preventive and effective against cell death. This would therefore limit brain degeneration.

## Improves Concentration

The ketones are a good source of fuel for the brain. As you decrease your carbohydrate intake, you avoid blood sugar spikes, which often appear after meals. This allows your body to avoid focusing on eliminating carbohydrates and to focus on the activity you are doing.

# Tips on Losing Weight After 50

## Learn How to Count Your Macros

This is especially important at the start of your journey. As time goes by, you will learn how to estimate your meals without using a food scale.

## Prepare Your Kitchen for Your Keto-friendly Foods

Once you've made a choice, it's time to get rid of all the foods in your kitchen that aren't allowed in the keto diet. To do this, check the nutritional labels of all the food items. Of course, there's no need to throw everything away. You can donate foods you don't need to food kitchens and other institutions that give food to the needy.

## Purchase Some Keto Strips for Yourself

These are important so you can check your ketone levels and track your progress. You can purchase keto strips in pharmacies and online. For instance, some of the best keto strips available on Amazon are Perfect Keto Ketone Test Strips, Smack fat Ketone Strips, and One Earth Ketone Strips.

## Find an Activity You Enjoy

When you have done enough exercise, you will know what activities you like. One way to encourage yourself to exercise more regularly is by making it entertaining than a chore. If possible, stick to your favorite activities, and you can get the most out of your exercises. Keep in mind that the activities you enjoy may not be effective or needed, so you need to find other exercises to compensate for, which you may not enjoy. For instance, if you like jogging, you can work your leg muscles, but your arms are not involved. So, you need to do pushups or other strength training exercises.

## Check with a Healthcare Provider

Your dietitian can tell you whether a keto diet would work. Still, it helps to check in with your healthcare provider to ensure that you do not have any medical condition that prevents you

KETO DIET AFTER 50

from losing weight, such as hypothyroidism and polycystic ovarian syndrome. It helps to know well in advance whether your body is even capable of losing fat in the first place before you commit and see no result, right?

## Hydrate Properly

That means drinking enough water or herbal tea and ditch sweetened beverages or other drinks that contain sugar altogether. Making the transition will be difficult for the first few weeks, but your body will be thanking you for it. There is nothing healthier than good old plain water, and the recommended amount is 2 gallons a day.

## Supplements

When you get older, your body starts to lose its ability to absorb certain nutrients, which leads to deficits. For example, vitamin B12 and folate are some of the most common nutrients that people over 50 lack. They have an impact on your mood, energy level, and weight loss rate.

## Have the Right Mindset

Your mindset is one of the most important things you need to change when you've decided to follow the keto lifestyle. Without the right mindset, you might not stick with the diet long enough to enjoy all its benefits. Also, the proper mindset will keep you motivated to keep going no matter what challenges come your way.

## Know Your Goals

It is sometimes helpful to remember what your goals are and why you want to meet those goals. This will be a good touchstone when you want to reach for a cookie or a sugary drink. Make sure you have that goal handy so that when you're feeling weak, you can remind yourself of your goals are and be determined to stick to them.

## Get Enough Sleep

Getting enough sleep helps your body regulate the hormones in your body, so try to aim for 7 to 9 hours of sleep a day. You can get more restful sleep by creating a nighttime routine that involves not looking at a computer, phone, or TV screen for at least 1 hour before bed. You can drink warm milk or water to help your body relax or even do 10 to 20 minutes of stretching to get a restful sleep.

## Keep a Food Log

Then add the calories and divide by three to get an average. Now that you know how many takes, you can figure out how much you need to pay on average per day to reach your goals.

## Ditch Those Carb-rich Foods Before You Start

There's nothing worse than feeling like you're comfortable on the Keto diet and super-happy with your progress, only to find a packet of potato chips or long-forgotten cheese fries lurking at the back of the pantry. Bang! There goes your willpower! Even if you have firm resolve, it's quite likely you'll succumb to temptation.

## Get Organized

The Organization is key to simplifying your Keto lifestyle, which helps you to stick to the diet. Plan your meals at the start of the week, organize a grocery list and go shopping ideally once to save you some time and energy.

## Make Sense of Eating Out

There's nothing worse than being 'that person' who can't eat a thing on the menu at a restaurant. So, do your homework!

Before you go anywhere, check out your local restaurants and find out if there's anything on the menu that will suit you. Check out the restaurants' online menus or pick up the phone and give them a call. It is fantastic to find your perfect restaurant; once you do, visit them often for your comfort.

## Avoid Sugary Liquids

Sugary drinks, ranging from energy drinks, your favorite soda, and fruit juices, are wealthy in unnecessary energy that increases your weight when you're looking to lose a few. The calories contained in sugary drinks are called negative energy. They do no longer have any nutritional blessings; they do no longer fill you, yet they nonetheless add for your body's caloric count.

Another aspect sugary liquid do is that because of the brought sugars, they increase your frame's tendency to store fats, especially in your abdomen.

## Eat Greater Veggies

Eating vegetables can never be under-envisioned because it has many benefits to the body. You can upload them on your meals, as lots of them are delicious. So, all you need to do is to eat a few delightful greens to lose weight.

## Consume Extra Culmination

Fruits are the second meals institution after veggies that you have to consume while seeking to shed pounds. Although some result is wealthy in sugar and shouldn't be eaten in high quantity, especially when on keto weight loss program and trying to lose weight, there are some extraordinary keto-friendly fruits you could eat.

## Control Your Quantities

It isn't news that the charge of our body's metabolism reduces each decade. So, once you recover from the age of 50, you could now not consume as you probably did for your teenage days. Therefore, consuming healthy foods is one of the most critical factors of dropping weight, even though being capable of manage portions is essential.

## Eat When You're Hungry

It is not a wholesome move to bypass out breakfast, mainly while you are attempting to lose a few weights. However, it is also very harmful to skip any meal while you get those starvation pangs. When you are hungry, it manner your body needs those vitamins but denying your body the vitamins isn't beneficial. Similar to skipping breakfast is skipping out any meal, which can also bring about binge consuming later.

# CHAPTER 4:

# Basic Fitness for the Ketogenic Diet

## The Importance of Exercise for People After 50

Exercising offers a plethora of benefits to all, regardless of your age! Healthy movement results in improved flexibility and stronger bones which is quite important for older folks. You see, as you age, your body's muscle mass starts to decrease. As we enter our forties, adults begin to lose three to five percent of muscle mass as they enter each new decade.

However, we do realize how the thought of exercising regularly at an older age can seem like a challenge, especially if you're feeling let down with frequent aches and pains. But in many ways, the benefits of exercising outweigh the potential risks. Let's dive into why exercising is so important for seniors.

## Benefits

Now, while you may be having thoughts about exercising, here are a couple of benefits that you can't ignore:

### Prevents Diseases

Regular physical activity has been known to reduce the risks of diseases such as diabetes and heart disease. This is mainly because exercise strengthens overall immune functioning which is particularly beneficial for seniors who are often immunocompromised. So even if you can't hit the gym some form of light exercise can play an integral role in disease management.

## Helps Increase Social Ties and Prevents Isolation

Aging can be a daunting process, but it becomes fun when you're surrounded by a community. Opting for yoga or fitness classes not only makes exercising more fun but it also helps you strengthen social ties with other older adults in your neighborhood. This can help ward off the occasional loneliness that one is likely to feel at old age. Plus, this will help you stay committed to your goals and lead a healthier lifestyle.

## Improves Cognitive Function

Regular exercise can also improve fine motor skills that boost cognitive function. Several studies have shown how exercising regularly can reduce the risk of dementia.

Unfortunately, older folks have a higher risk of falling which can lead to dangerous injuries. This can also drastically reduce your chances of leading an independent life as you grow older. As seniors take much longer to recover from injuries and falls, it is important to exercise to improve balance add mobility.

# Simple Exercises for Seniors

Here is a list of simple exercises that people in their fifties and beyond can enjoy:

## Light Weight Training

You can start off with a little weight training to retain bone density and build muscle mass. If you're more interested in doing home exercises than joining the gym, invest in 2-pound weights, and perform arm raises and shoulder presses.

Ideally, we recommend that you join a fitness center or gym where you can meet like-minded folks. You can also get yourself a personal trainer who can recommend customized workouts for you. Either way, remember to take it slow at first as you don't want to exert yourself too much.

## Walking

If lifting weights isn't for you, good old-fashioned walking should also work for you. Consider taking a nice walk around your neighborhood or go to a park nearby. You'll be able to make some friends and enjoy the weather while you're at it too.

In case you'd rather workout at home, strap on a pedometer, and get going around the house. You'll be able to get more out of this workout if you move your arms and lift your knees as you take each step.

## Aerobics

Joining an aerobics class can significantly help you keep your muscles strong whilst maintaining mobility. This will not only improve balance but will reduce the risk of falls, thus drastically improving the overall quality of your life as you grow older.

Many studies have also indicated how aerobic exercises can protect memory and sharpen your mind and improving cognitive function among older adults. If you're not comfortable joining a class, you'll find plenty of videos online. Aerobic exercises have also been known to get the heart pumping, improving cardiovascular help.

## Swimming

Do you find regular exercise too boring? Swimming is a fun, impact-free exercise that can get yours through the day. It's almost pain-free and won't trouble your aging joints. Swimming offers resistance training and will help you get back up to your feet again.

Here's how it works: the water offers gentle resistance while giving you a cardiovascular workout too. This also builds muscle capacity and helps you build strength too.

## Yoga

What's no to love about yoga? It's relaxing, it's healthy and you can enjoy it with a group. Yoga does an excellent job of improving flexibility in your joints. It allows seniors to remain limber and maintain their sense of balance. If you have trouble moving about or stretching, then you can try chair yoga.

Some classic yoga poses that you might want to try out include seated forward bend, downward facing dog, and warrior.

## Squats

When you're working on an exercise program, you shouldn't skip the idea of strength training. Squats happen to be an excellent way to strengthen the muscles of your lower body. Doing squats is relatively easy and you won't need any sort of equipment except for maybe a chair to support yourself. However, if you have trouble with balance, we suggest you skip this exercise and opt for something much simpler.

## Sit-Ups

Sit-ups are a great way to strengthen your core muscles, improve back pain problems, and balance. Performing simple sit-ups should do the job. All you have to do is lie down on your back and keep your knees bent at an angle. Now place your hands behind your head and then gently try to lift your head. You should feel the sensation in your core muscles.

## Light cardio

Specific aerobic exercises are perfect for you if you are just getting started on keto, although you have to keep them at low intensity (a maximum heart rate of 40-50%). The following cardiovascular workouts can help you ease into keto diet while you adapt to it:

- swimming

- hiking

- rowing

- biking

## Simple resistance workouts

Many people often believe that you need carbs to build muscle, but this is not true. It does not matter if you are adapted to keto or not. As far as you eat enough protein, you will be able to build strength and lean mass with ketones serving as fuel. You can try some light weightlifting as you transit into the keto diet.

# How Keto Impacts Your Exercise Performance

Your cells produce energy for your body by making use of two primary energy sources, which include fatty acids and glucose. As I said earlier, ketosis is a state where your body uses fatty acids predominantly as a source of energy through a process known as beta-oxidation. When you start dieting, your body makes more use of fatty acid to generate energy. However, this shift takes time for your body to adapt to it.

During this time, the body experiences the keto flu (because of the adjustment period), and sleep and irritability problems may arise. You might be experiencing the keto flu because of the following reasons:

1. Your body needs time to adapt to the keto diet

2. Micronutrients and electrolyte are deficient

3. Withdrawal from carbs that have the same symptoms with caffeine withdrawal occurs

# Making Keto and Exercising a Perfect Match

If you are just getting started on a keto diet, and you want to engage in some high intensity, it is essential to know the version of the keto diet that is appropriate for you. One of the best things about keto is that it can be modified, depending on your needs. This ability to adapt the keto diet to your needs in combination with your workout routine goes a long way in giving you a healthy life.

# Things You Need to Know Before Exercising

## The First Stage is the Hardest

Even without you being a woman of 50 years, the first weeks of exercise while on the keto diet is always the hardest. As your body learns or adapts to using ketones as a source of energy, you will feel less energetic than usual, and this is especially apparent when you begin workouts.

According to the results of some research, while you might find the initial stages of exercises on keto diet hard, it does get better with time. An Associate Professor of Neurology based in New York at the Weill Cornell Medical Center started studying how keto diets affect our performance during exercise. In his research published in the Journal of the International Society of Sports Nutrition in July 2017, he said that while people on keto diet might experience reduced energy initially when beginning the workout. However, people on keto diet might find it difficult to undergo exercises of higher intensity.

Another reason why one feels very sluggish during the first periods of workout is the low carb content of a diet. Your muscles store glycogen used for quick energy generation. The low carb content of keto diets causes the glycogen stores of the muscles to be depleted. This leaves your body with just fat to use for energy, and fat isn't as readily available as carbs.

To adapt correctly for exercising while on the keto diet, you need to focus on workouts that rely on fat as a source of fuel. You can go with a low-intensity workout or cardio, which uses more fat as a source of fuel rather than high-intensity exercises that use sugar as a source of fuel.

## How to Overcome the First Stage?

### The Type of Workout Matters

Although in the first stage, you may find it challenging to carry out many high-intensity workouts such as sprinting, weightlifting, or another exercise that requires a quick boost of energy, you can still be able to carry out the low-intensity activity. Even after the first few weeks of workouts, strenuous exercises will always be difficult. Therefore, it is essential to adjust the workouts to go in line with your nutrition.

You might want to change your mind on your favorite HIIT (high-intensity workouts)

During a workout, you will notice that you get tired quicker than usual. Mainly, during the first stages of exercise on the keto diet, you will find out you have a low endurance level. This does not mean that you should give up on a workout. Low-intensity workouts are the best way to go. Low-intensity exercises such as jogging, bike riding, and yoga are more natural for the body. This low-intensity exercise is the best during the first two to three weeks of workouts on the keto diet.

So, instead of going for that sprinting weightlifting or any workouts that add extra stress, just take it easy and let your body adjust. One of the benefits of working out on the keto diet is that it leads to an increase in lean body mass. Several studies have shown that working out on keto diet helps in losing body weight; it increases lean body mass at the same time.

You might want to switch things up if you are struggling with the keto diet and exercising

If you always feel drained during workout while on the standard keto diet, you could try out another variant of the keto diet, named a cyclical ketogenic diet (also known as keto cycling). Choosing this alternative, you go with the standard keto diet for most of the week. Then, you dedicate one or two meals with higher carb content to restore energy levels. However, it is fundamental to note that you might kick your body out of ketosis on the days you eat more carbs.

## Listen to Your Body When Mixing Keto and Engaging in Exercise

This is especially important during the first few weeks. If you often end up feeling tired and dizzy, your body may not be working well on a low-carb diet. Your health and wellbeing should always come first. You could add some carbs to your diet to see if you feel better. If you do feel better, then you might want to tweak things a little to balance the needs of your body.

# How Exercises While on Keto Boost Your Performance

If you are just getting started on a keto diet, then you have taken a good step towards:

- Having a better body composition

- Lesser inflammation

- High level of energy

But exercise is essential too. An inactive and sedentary lifestyle is associated with a lot of chronic diseases like obesity and diabetes. A regular exercise routine helps in:

- Burning fat

- Building your strength

- Improving your body's composition

- Improving your mood (during a workout, the adrenaline released helps to burn fat as it travels to your brain, thereby making you happier)

- Making your workouts more effective so that when you are advanced in age, with the keto diet, you are still going to get the most out of your workouts

An example is seen in early humans. They didn't have the opportunity to eat foods rich in carbs despite that their performance needed to be high during long hunting periods.

Studies have shown that the keto diet enhances performance while working out

Athletes on keto diets burned 2-3 times fatter than those on high carb

In a more recent study, athletes performing endurance workouts burned more fats and recovered faster after ten weeks while on keto

After several weeks on keto, obese individuals were able to walk on a treadmill almost twice

Cyclists on the keto diet lost more fat than those who were on placebo-fed controls

Young men on keto added more muscle mass weightlifting than those on a high-carb diet

In some of these researches, the participants were given enough time to adapt to the keto diet and ketosis. However, if you are just getting started and you are still in the process of adjusting to using fat as fuel, then here are some excellent exercises for beginners.

# CHAPTER 5:

# Four-Week Keto Meal Plan

| DAYS | BREAKFAST | LUNCH | DINNER |
|---|---|---|---|
| 1 | Indian Chicken Curry | Fennel Quiche | Keto Summer Options |
| 2 | Persian Chicken | Turkey Hash | Keto Coleslaw Stuffed Wraps |
| 3 | Pesto Pork Chops | Lemon Salmon and Broccoli Casserole | Keto Dried Beef & Cream Cheese Ball |
| 4 | Slow Cooker Brisket | Herbed Shrimp with Cilantro | Keto Smoked Salmon Wraps |
| 5 | Garlic Beef Stir-Fry | Indian Chicken Curry | Fennel Quiche |
| 6 | Pumpkin and Beef Sautée | Persian Chicken | Turkey Hash |
| 7 | Crispy Chicken Drumsticks | Pesto Pork Chops | Lemon Salmon and Broccoli Casserole |
| 8 | Chicken Fillet with Brussels Sprouts | Slow Cooker Brisket | Herbed Shrimp with Cilantro |

| 9 | Indian Beef | Garlic Beef Stir-Fry | Indian Chicken Curry |
|---|---|---|---|
| 10 | Seafood - Coconut Stew | Pumpkin and Beef Sautée | Persian Chicken |
| 11 | Simple "Grilled" Shrimp | Crispy Chicken Drumsticks | Pesto Pork Chops |
| 12 | Mussels ala Marinera | Chicken Fillet with Brussels Sprouts | Slow Cooker Brisket |
| 13 | Creamy Chicken Salad | Indian Beef | Garlic Beef Stir-Fry |
| 14 | Spicy Keto Chicken Wings | Seafood - Coconut Stew | Pumpkin and Beef Sautée |
| 15 | Cheesy Ham Quiche | Simple "Grilled" Shrimp | Crispy Chicken Drumsticks |
| 16 | Baked Cod with Cucumber-Dill Salsa | Mussels ala Marinera | Chicken Fillet with Brussels Sprouts |
| 17 | Roasted Red Pepper and Eggplant Soup | Creamy Chicken Salad | Seafood - Coconut Stew |
| 18 | Cilantro-Lime Flounder | Spicy Keto Chicken Wings | Indian Beef |
| 19 | Seafood Casserole | Cheesy Ham Quiche | Simple "Grilled" Shrimp |

| 20 | Sausage Omelet | Baked Cod with Cucumber-Dill Salsa | Mussels ala Marinera |
|---|---|---|---|
| 21 | Brown Hash with Zucchini | Roasted Red Pepper and Eggplant Soup | Creamy Chicken Salad |
| 22 | Crunchy Radish & Zucchini Hash Browns | Cilantro-Lime Flounder | Spicy Keto Chicken Wings |
| 23 | Keto Bacon Guacamole Fat Bombs | Seafood Casserole | Cheesy Ham Quiche |
| 24 | Keto Salmon & Cream Cheese Bites | Sausage Omelet | Baked Cod with Cucumber-Dill Salsa |
| 25 | Keto Summer Options | Brown Hash with Zucchini | Roasted Red Pepper and Eggplant Soup |
| 26 | Keto Coleslaw Stuffed Wraps | Crunchy Radish & Zucchini Hash Browns | Cilantro-Lime Flounder |
| 27 | Keto Dried Beef & Cream Cheese Ball | Keto Bacon Guacamole Fat Bombs | Seafood Casserole |
| 28 | Keto Smoked Salmon Wraps | Keto Salmon & Cream Cheese Bites | Sausage Omelet |

# CHAPTER 6:

# Keto Recipes - The Top 30 Recipes

## Indian Chicken Curry

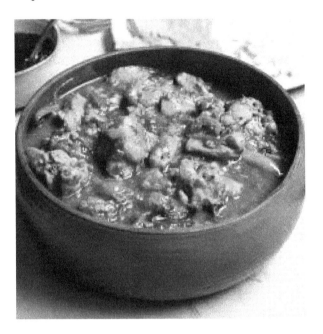

**Preparation Time**: 20 minutes

**Cooking Time**: 40 minutes

**Servings**: 6

**Ingredients:**

- 3 tablespoons of olive oil, divided

- 6 boneless, skinless chicken thighs

- 1 small sweet onion

- 2 tablespoons of fresh garlic

- 1 tablespoon of fresh ginger

- 1 tablespoon of Hot Curry Powder

- ¾ cup of water

- ¼ cup of coconut milk

- 2 tablespoons of fresh cilantro.

## Directions

1. Place 2 tablespoons of oil over medium to a high place in a large skillet.

2. Add the chicken and roast for about 10 minutes until the thighs are browned all over.

3. Remove the chicken on a plate with tongs and set aside.

4. In the skillet, add the remaining 1 tablespoon of oil and sauté the onion, garlic, and ginger for about 3 minutes or until softened.

5. Remove the curry powder, water, and milk from the coconut.

6. Go back to the skillet with the chicken and bring the liquid to a boil.

7. Reduce heat to low, cover the skillet and cook for 26 minutes or until the chicken is tender and the sauce is thick. Serve with cilantro on hand.

# Persian Chicken

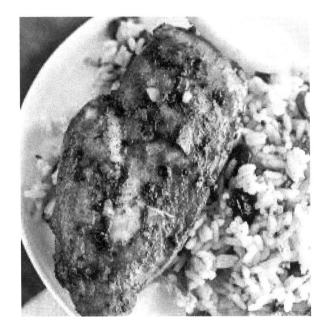

**Preparation Time**: 10 minutes

**Cooking Time**: 20 minutes

**Servings**: 6

**Ingredients:**

- ½ small sweet onion,

- ¼ cup freshly squeezed lemon juice

- 1 tablespoon dried oregano

- 1/2 tablespoon of sweet paprika,

- ½ tablespoon of ground cumin

- ½ cup olive oil

- 6 boneless, skinless chicken thighs

## Directions:

1. Put the vegetables in a blender. Mix it well.

2. Put the olive while the motor is running.

3. In a sealable bag for the freezer, place the chicken thighs and put the mixture in the sealable bag.

4. Refrigerate it for 2 hours, while turning it two times.

5. Remove the marinade thighs and discard the additional marinade. Preheat to medium the barbecue. Grill the chicken, turning once or until the internal

# Pesto Pork Chops

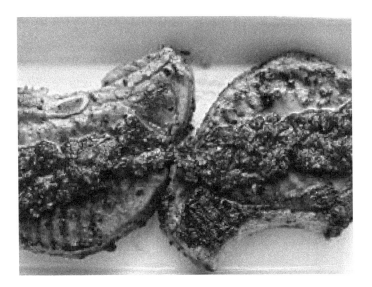

Preparation **Time**: 20 minutes

**Cooking Time**: 20 minutes

**Servings**: 3

**Ingredients**:

- 3(3-ounce) top-flood pork chops, boneless, fat

- 8 tablespoons Herb Pesto (here)

- ½ cup breadcrumbs

- 1 tablespoon olive oil

**Directions**:

1. Preheat the oven to 360 ° F. Cover a foil baker's sheet; set aside.

2. Rub 1 tablespoon of pesto evenly across each pork chop on both sides.

3. Every pork chop in the crumbs of bread is lightly dredged.

4. Heat the oil in a medium-high heat large skillet. Brown the pork chops for about 6 minutes on each side.

5. Place the pork chops on the baking sheet. Bake until the pork reaches 136 ° F in the center for about 10 minutes.

# Slow Cooker Brisket

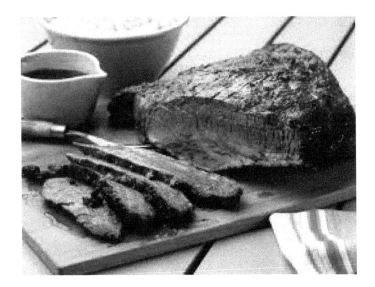

**Preparation and Cooking time**: 6 hours and 10 minutes

**Servings**: 6

**Ingredients**:

- 1 bottle Lager beer

- 3 lb. Beef brisket

- 0.25 teaspoon Pepper

- 0.5 teaspoon Salt

- 0.5 teaspoon Cumin

- 0.5 teaspoon Smoked paprika

- 1 teaspoon Instant coffee crystals

- 1 tablespoon Brown sugar

**Directions:**

1. Take out a bowl and combine the pepper, salt, cumin, paprika, coffee crystals, and brown sugar.

2. Using your hands, you can rub this mixture all over the brisket. Be sure to coat evenly

3. Set the slow cooker to a high setting before adding the brisket inside.

4. Pour the beer all over the brisket and then place the lid on top of the slow cooker.

5. Cover the slow cooker and cook it on high for about 6 hours. When the brisket is done, allow it to cool for about 10 minutes. Then slice or shred up the meat in 6 pieces before serving.

# Garlic Beef Stir-Fry

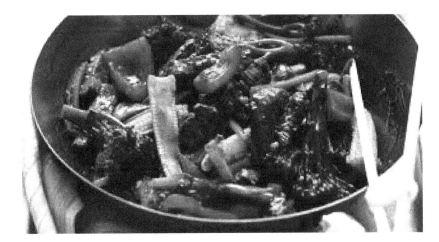

**Preparation and Cooking time**: 35 minutes

**Servings**: 6

**Ingredients**:

- 1 lb. lean beef strips

- 2 cloves garlic, crushed

- 1 tablespoon sweet chili sauce (homemade preferred)

- 21 oz. stir-fried vegetable mix

- ¼ cup water

- 2 tablespoons oyster sauce

**Directions**:

1. Set greased wok over high heat. Stir-fry beef in batches until almost cooked. Transfer to a plate and set aside.

2. Stir-fry the vegetables, garlic, and chili sauce until the veggies are tender.

3. Return the beef to the wok. Add water and oyster sauce. Continue to cook until it simmers.

4. Transfer to a serving plate and serve.

# Pumpkin and Beef Sautée

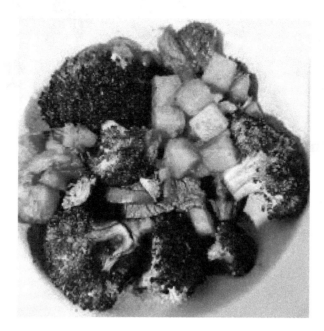

**Preparation and Cooking time**: 45 minutes

**Servings:** 6

**Ingredients**:

- 1.76 lbs. grass-fed beef, minced

- 8.8 oz. organic bacon, sliced into strips

  - lbs. pumpkin, peeled, seeded, and diced

- tablespoon ghee, divided

- 3-4 tablespoons fresh parsley, chopped

- ½ teaspoon cayenne pepper

- 1 tablespoon paprika

- ¼ teaspoon sea salt

- Pinch freshly ground black pepper

## Directions:

1. Transfer beef to a bowl and let it rest at room temperature.

2. Meanwhile, grease the pan with 2 tablespoon of ghee and transfer the pumpkin cubes. Season the pumpkin with salt and cover the pan with a lid. Cook over low-medium heat for about 10 minutes. Stir once or twice to avoid burning.

3. Meanwhile, set another pan over medium heat and roast the bacon until brown. Set aside.

4. Season the beef with spices (black pepper, paprika, and cayenne) and salt.

5. Grease another pan with the remaining ghee and brown the beef. Stir frequently to avoid burning.

6. Once the beef is done, add the bacon and remove the pan from the heat. Add the parsley.

7. Once the pumpkin is done, add it to the beef mixture. Mix until well-incorporated.

8. Serve and enjoy!

# Crispy Chicken Drumsticks

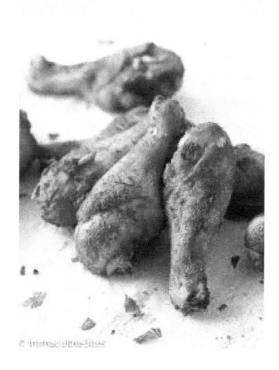

**Preparation and cooking time**: 50 minutes

**Servings**: 6

## Ingredients

- 4 chicken drumsticks

- 1 teaspoon dried basil

- 1 teaspoon dried oregano

- 1 tablespoon olive oil

- 1 teaspoon paprika

- Salt, to your liking

## Directions

1   Pat dry the chicken drumsticks and rub them with olive oil, salt, black pepper, paprika, basil, and oregano.

2   Preheat your oven to 410 degrees F. Coat a baking pan with a piece of parchment paper.

3   Bake the chicken drumsticks until they are browned on all sides for 40 to 45 minutes.

# Chicken Fillet with Brussels Sprouts

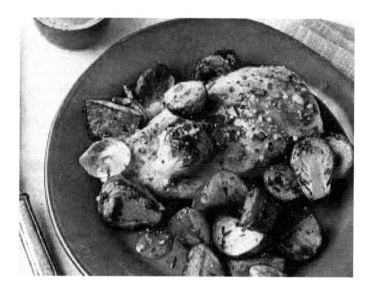

**Preparation and cooking time:** 20 minutes

**Servings:** 6

**Ingredients:**

- 3/4-pound chicken breasts, chopped into bite-sized pieces

- 1/2 teaspoon ancho Chile powder

- 1/2 teaspoon whole black peppercorns

- 1/2 cup onions, chopped

- cup vegetable broth

- tablespoons olive oil

- 1/4 teaspoon garlic salt

- clove garlic, minced

- tablespoons port wine

**Directions:**

1. Heat 1 tablespoon of the oil in a frying pan over medium-high heat. Sauté the Brussels sprouts for about 3 minutes or until golden on all sides. Salt to taste and reserve.

2. Heat the remaining tablespoon of olive oil—Cook the garlic and chicken for about 3 minutes.

3. Add in the onions, vegetable broth, wine, Ancho Chile powder, and black peppercorns; bring to a boil. Then, reduce the temperature to simmer and continue to cook for 4 to 5 minutes longer.

4. Add the reserved Brussels sprouts back to the frying pan.

# Indian Beef

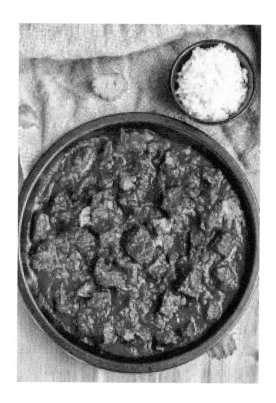

**Preparation and Cooking Time**: 35 minutes

**Servings**: 6

**Ingredients**:

- ½ tablespoon olive oil

- ¼ yellow onion, chopped

- garlic clove, minced

- ½ jalapeño pepper, chopped

- ½ pound grass-fed ground beef

- ½ cup cherry tomatoes, quartered

- ½ pound fresh collard greens, trimmed and chopped

- ½ teaspoon fresh lemon juice

## Spices

- ½ teaspoon ground coriander

- ½ teaspoon ground cumin

- ¼ teaspoon ground fennel seeds

- ¼ teaspoon ground ginger

- ¼ teaspoon ground cinnamon

- ¼ teaspoon ground turmeric

- Salt and black pepper, to taste

## Directions:

1. Put olive oil and onions in a skillet and sauté for about 5 minutes.

2. Add garlic and jalapeno and sauté for about 1 minute.

3. Add beef and spices and cook for about 10 minutes, continuously stirring.

4. Stir in tomatoes and collard greens and cook for about 4 minutes.

5. Add lemon juice, salt and black pepper and dish out to serve.

6. You can refrigerate it by placing it in containers for meal prepping purpose and refrigerate it up to 4 days. Reheat in microwave when you want to use it again.

# Seafood - Coconut Stew

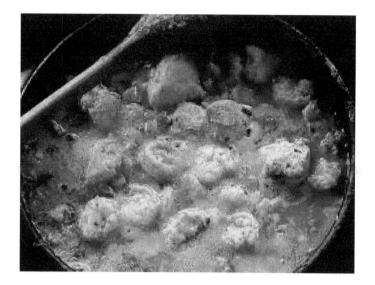

**Preparation Time**: 10 minutes

**Cooking Time**:2 minutes

**Servings**: 6

**Ingredients:**

- 1 lb white fish fillet

- 2 pinch of sea salt

- 2 cloves garlic, finely chopped

- 1 tablespoon coriander fresh, finely chopped

- 1 lemon juice, freshly squeezed

- 2 tablespoons olive oil

- 2 spring onions finely chopped

- 1 grated tomato

- 1 lb of shrimp

- 2 cups of coconut milk

- 1 cup water

## Directions:

1. Season the fish with salt, garlic, coriander, and lemon juice.

2. Pour olive oil in your Instant Pot and layer the fish fillets.

3. Put chopped onions, tomatoes and peppers and sprinkle with a coriander on top.

4. Pour 1/2 cup water.

5. Lock lid into place and set on the MANUAL setting for 2 minutes.

6. When the timer beeps, press "Cancel" and carefully flip the Quick Release valve to let the pressure out.

7. Open the lid and add shrimps and coconut milk: stir to combine well.

8. Lock lid into place and set on the MANUAL setting for 1 minute.

9. Use Quick Release - turn the valve from sealing to venting to release the pressure.

10. Serve hot.

## Simple "Grilled" Shrimp

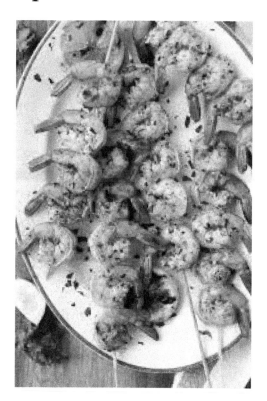

**Preparation Time**: 10 minutes

**Cooking Time:**2 minutes

**Servings**: 6

**Ingredients**:

- 2 tablespoons fresh butter softened

- 1 1/2 lb shrimp 21-25 size, peeled, deveined

- Sea-salt flakes

- 1 tablespoon fresh tarragon and chervil finely chopped

- 1 cup water

- Lemon wedges for serving

**Directions**:

1. Add the butter to the inner stainless-steel pot in the Instant Pot.

2. Add shrimp into Instant Pot, and sprinkle with sea-salt flakes and chopped tarragon and chervil.

3. Lock lid into place and set on the MANUAL setting for 2 minutes.

4. When the timer beeps, press "Cancel" and carefully flip the Quick Release valve to let the pressure out.

5. Ready! Serve with lemon wedges.

# Mussels ala Marinera

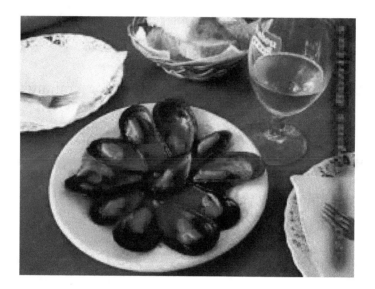

**Preparation Time:** 15 minutes

**Cooking Time:**3 hours

**Servings**: 6

**Ingredients**:

- lbs. of mussels, cleaned

- 1 small onions, chopped

- 1 tablespoon of ground paprika

- 2 tablespoons of almond flour

- 1 glass of white wine

- 1 cup of bone broth

- A bunch of chopped fresh parsley

- Salt to taste

- 2 tablespoons of extra virgin olive oil

- bay leaves

**Directions**:

1. Place the mussels in your Slow Cooker along with all remaining ingredients.

2. Cover and cook on HIGH for 2 hours.

3. Open lid removes mussels; debeard and clean them.

4. Place mussels in a Slow Cooker, cover and cook on HIGH for further 1 hour.

5. Serve.

# Creamy Chicken Salad

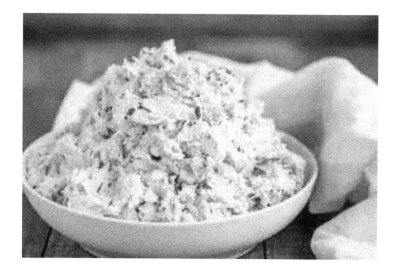

**Preparation Time:** 10 minutes

**Cooking Time**: 30 minutes

**Servings**: 4

**Ingredients**:

- Chicken Breast - 1 Lb.

- Avocado - 2

- Garlic Cloves - 2,

- Minced Lime Juice - 3 T.

- Onion - .33 C.,

- Minced Jalapeno Pepper - 1,

- Minced Salt - Dash Cilantro - 1 T.

- Pepper - Dash

## Directions

1. You will want to start this recipe off my prepping the stove to 400. As this warms up, get out your cooking sheet and line it with paper or foil.

2. Next, it is time to get out of the chicken.

3. Go ahead and layer the chicken breast up with some olive oil before seasoning to your liking.

4. When the chicken is all set, you will want to line them along the surface of your cooking sheet and pop it into the oven for about twenty minutes.

5. By the end of twenty minutes, the chicken should be cooked through and can be taken out of the oven for chilling.

6. Once cool enough to handle, you will want to either dice or shred your chicken, dependent upon how you like your chicken salad.

7. Now that your chicken is all cooked, it is time to assemble your salad!

8. You can begin this process by adding everything into a bowl and mashing down the avocado.

9. Once your ingredients are mended to your liking, sprinkle some salt over the top and serve immediately.

## Spicy Keto Chicken Wings

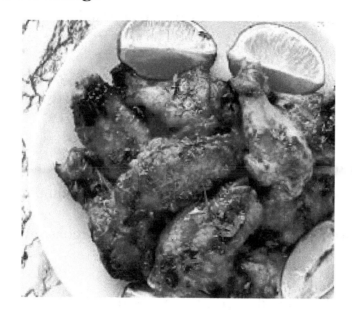

**Preparation Time**: 20 minutes

**Cooking Time**: 30 minutes

**Servings**: 4

**Ingredients:**

- Chicken Wings - 2 Lbs.

- Cajun Spice - 1 tablespoon.

- Smoked Paprika - 2 tablespoon.

- Turmeric - .50 tablespoon.

- Salt - Dash

- Baking Powder - 2 tablespoon.

- Pepper - Dash

**Directions:**

1.  When you first begin the Ketogenic Diet, you may find that you won't be eating the traditional foods that may have made up a majority of your diet in the past.

2.  While this is a good thing for your health, you may feel you are missing out! The good news is that there are delicious alternatives that aren't lacking in flavor! To start this recipe, you'll want to prep the stove to 400.

3.  As this heat up, you will want to take some time to dry your chicken wings with a paper towel. This will help remove any excess moisture and get you some nice, crispy wings!

4.  When you are all set, take out a mixing bowl and place all of the seasonings along with the baking powder. If you feel like it, you can adjust the seasoning levels however you would like.

5.  Once these are set, go ahead, and throw the chicken wings in and coat evenly. If you have one, you'll want to place the wings on a wire rack that is placed over your baking tray. If not, you can just lay them across the baking sheet.

6.  Now that your chicken wings are set, you are going to pop them into the stove for thirty minutes. By the end of this time, the tops of the wings should be crispy.

7.  If they are, take them out from the oven and flip them so that you can bake the other side. You will want to cook these for an additional thirty minutes.

8.  Finally, take the tray from the oven and allow it to cool slightly before serving up your spiced keto wings. For additional flavor, serve with any of your favorite, keto-friendly dipping sauce.

# Cheesy Ham Quiche

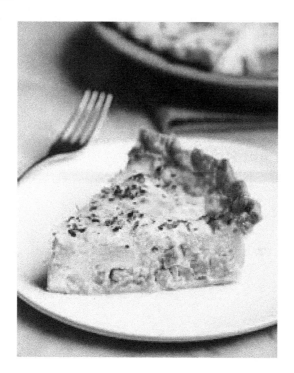

**Preparation Time**: 10 minutes

**Cooking Time:** 30 minutes

**Servings**: 6

**Ingredients:**

- Eggs - 8

- Zucchini - 1 C.,

- Shredded heavy Cream - .50 C.

- Ham - 1 C., Diced

- Mustard - 1 tsp.

- Salt – Dash

**Directions:**

1. For this recipe, you can start by prepping your stove to 375 and getting out a pie plate for your quiche.

2. Next, it is time to prep the zucchini. First, you will want to go ahead and shred it into small pieces.

3. Once this is complete, take a paper towel and gently squeeze out the excess moisture. This will help avoid a soggy quiche.

4. When the step from above is complete, you will want to place the zucchini into your pie plate along with the cooked ham pieces and your cheese.

5. Once these items are in place, you will want to whisk the seasonings, cream, and eggs together before pouring it over the top.

6. Now that your quiche is set, you are going to pop the dish into your stove for about forty minutes.

7. By the end of this time, the egg should be cooked through, and you will be able to insert a knife into the center and have it come out clean.

8. If the quiche is cooked to your liking, take the dish from the oven, and allow it to chill slightly before slicing and serving.

# Baked Cod with Cucumber-Dill Salsa

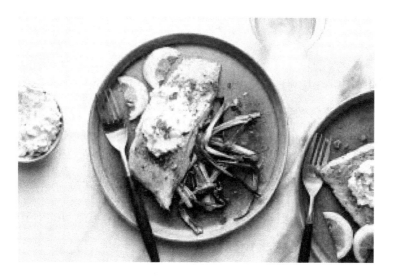

**Preparation Time:** 20 minutes

**Cooking Time**: 10 minutes

**Servings**: 3

**Ingredients:**

**For the cucumber salsa:**

- ½ English cucumber, diced

- 2 teaspoons of fresh dill Juice of 1 lime Zest of 1 lime

- ¼ cup of boiling red pepper

- ½ teaspoon of granulated sugar

**For the fish:**

- ounces of cod fillets, deboned and divided into 3 parts

- Juice of 1 lemon

- ½ tablespoon of freshly ground black pepper

- 1 tablespoon of olive oil

**Directions**:

1. In a small bowl, combine the cucumber.

2. Preheat the oven to 360 degrees F. Place the fish on a pie plate and squeeze the juice over the fillets evenly.

3. Sprinkle over the fillets evenly with pepper and drizzle the olive oil. Bake the fish with a fork for about 6 minutes or until it easily flakes.

4. Transfer the fish to 3 plates and serve on top with the salsa of cucumber.

5. Modification of dialysis:

6. Try this baked fish with a sprinkling of fresh dill and a bit of lime zest instead of salsa to reduce the amount of potassium.

# Roasted Red Pepper and Eggplant Soup

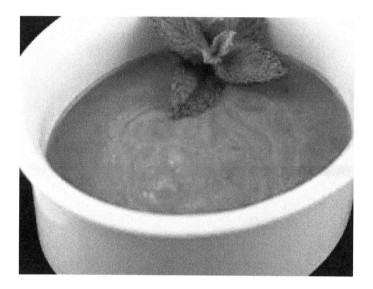

**Preparation Time:** 20 minutes

**Cooking Time**: 40 minutes

**Servings**: 6

**Ingredients**:

- 1 small sweet onion, cut into quarters

- 2 small red peppers, halved

- 2 cups of eggplant

- 2 garlic cloves, crushed

- 1 cup of olive oil

- 1 cup of Easy Chicken Stock (here)

- Water

- ¼ cup of chopped fresh basil

**Directions:**

1. Preheat the oven to 360 ° F. In a large ovenproof baking dish, place the onions, red peppers, eggplant, and garlic.

2. Add the olive oil to the vegetables.

3. For about 40 minutes or until slightly charred and soft, roast the vegetables.

4. Slightly cool the vegetables and remove the peppers from the skin.

5. In a food processor (or in a large bowl, using a handheld immersion blender) purée the vegetables with the chicken stock.

6. Move the soup to a large pot and add sufficient water to achieve the desired thickness. Heat the soup and add the basil to a simmer. Season and serve with pepper.

# Cilantro-Lime Flounder

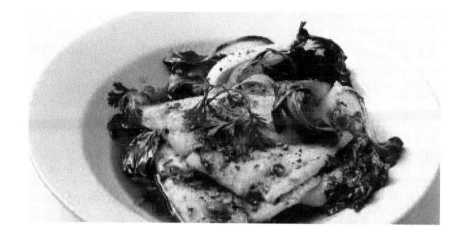

**Preparation Time:** 20 minutes

**Cooking Time**: 6 minutes

**Servings**: 3

**Ingredients:**

- ¼ cup homemade mayonnaise (here)

- 1 lime juice Zest

- 1 ½ cup fresh cilantro

- 3(3-ounce) flounder fillets

**Directions**:

1. Preheat the oven to 300 ° F. Stir the mayonnaise, lime juice, lime zest, and cilantro in a small bowl.

2. Place 3 pieces of foil on a clean work surface, about 8 by 8 inches square. In the center of each square, place a flounder fillet.

3. Top the fillets with the mixture of mayonnaise evenly.

4. Season the pepper to the flounder. Fold the foil sides over the fish, create a snug packet, and place on a baking sheet the foil packets.

5. Bake the fish for three to six minutes.

6. Unfold and display the boxes.

# Seafood Casserole

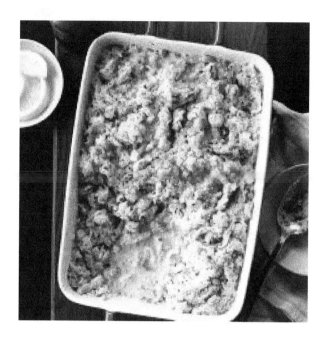

**Preparation Time**: 20 minutes

**Cooking Time**: 36 minutes

**Servings**: 6

**Ingredients**:

- 2 cups of eggplant,

- Sliced and cut in 1-inch bits of butter,

- 1 tablespoon of olive oil

- ½ small sweet onion,

- 1 tablespoon of minced garlic

- 1 celery stalk,

- ½ red bell pepper,

- tablespoons of freshly squeezed lemon juice

- 1 tablespoon of hot sauce

- ¼ tablespoon of Creole Seasoning Mix (here)

- ½ cup of white rice,

- 1 large egg

- 3 ounces of cooked shrimp.

## Directions:

1. Cook the eggplant for 6 minutes in a small saucepan filled with water over medium-high heat. Drain in a large bowl and set aside.

2. Grease and set aside an 8-by-13-inch butter baking dish. Heat the olive oil in a large pot over medium heat.

3. Drizzle the onion, garlic, celery, and pepper bell for about 3 minutes or until tender. In addition to the lemon juice, hot sauce, Creole seasoning, rice, and egg, add the sautéed vegetables to the eggplant.

4. Remove to combine. Fold in the meat of the crab and shrimp.

5. In the casserole dish, spoon the casserole mixture and pat down the top. Bake for 26 to 40 minutes until the casserole is heated through and the rice is tender. Serve hot.

## Sausage Omelet

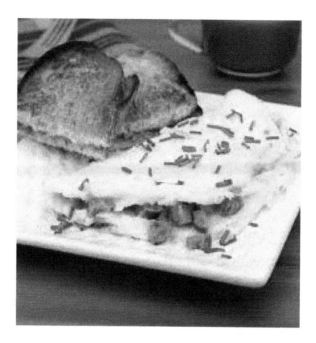

**Preparation Time**: 20 minutes

**Cooking Time**: 30 minutes

**Servings**: 6

**Ingredients**:

- ½ pound gluten-free sausage links, casing removed and crumbled

- ½ cup heavy whipping cream

- Salt and black pepper, to taste

- large organic eggs

- 1 cup cheddar cheese, shredded

- ¼ tsp. red pepper flakes, crushed

**Directions**:

1. Preheat your oven to 350°F. Grease a 9x13-inch baking dish. Heat a nonstick frying pan over medium heat and cook the sausage for about 8–10 minutes or until cooked through.

2. Meanwhile, in a bowl, add the remaining ingredients and beat until well combined. Remove from the heat and drain off the grease completely.

3. Place cooked sausage in the bottom of prepared baking dish evenly and top with the egg mixture.

4. Bake for approximately 30 minutes or until eggs are completely set.

5. Remove from oven and carefully transfer the omelet onto a cutting board. Cut into desired-sized wedges and serve.

# Brown Hash with Zucchini

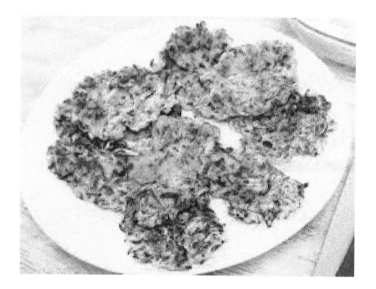

**Preparation Time:** 20 minutes

**Cooking Time**: 30 minutes

**Servings**: 6

**Ingredients**:

- 1 Sliced small onion

- to 8 medium sliced mushrooms

- 2 Cups of grass-fed ground beef

- 1 Pinch of salt

- 1 Pinch of ground black pepper

- ½ tsp of smoked paprika

- 2 Lightly beaten eggs

- 1 Small diced avocado

- Sliced pitted black olives

## Directions:

1. Preheat your air fryer to a temperature of about 350° F. Spray your air fryer pan with a little bit of melted coconut oil.

2. Add the onions, the mushrooms, the salt, and the pepper to the pan. Add the ground beef and the smoked paprika and crack in the eggs.

3. Gently whisk your mixture; then place the pan in your Air Fryer and lock the lid. Set the timer to about 18 to 20 minutes and the temperature to about 375° F.

4. When the timer beeps; turn off your Air Fryer; then remove the pan from the Air Fryer.

5. Serve and enjoy your breakfast with chopped parsley and diced avocado!

# Crunchy Radish & Zucchini Hash Browns

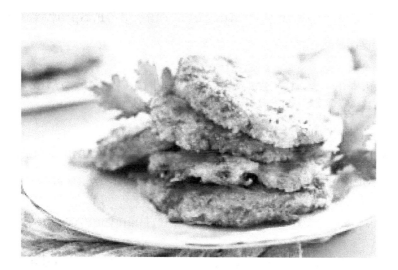

**Preparation Time**: 20 minutes

**Cooking Time**: 40 minutes

**Servings**: 6

**Ingredients**:

- 1 teaspoon onion powder

- 1/2 cup zucchini, shredded, drained

- 1/ cup cheese (cheddar), shredded

- 1/2 cup radishes, riced

- egg whites

- Pepper & salt to taste

**Directions:**

1. Stir in the radishes, zucchini, seasonings, and cheese. Shape into 6 patties. Heat your skillet over medium-high flame heat.

2. Drizzle with some olive oil. Sear each side of the patties till brown.

3. Reduce the heat to medium-low; cook for 3 to 5 minutes more.

4. To bake, preheat your oven to 425F. Oil a muffin tin, pack the mixture into each cup. Bake for 15 minutes or till brown and set.

## Keto Bacon Guacamole Fat Bombs

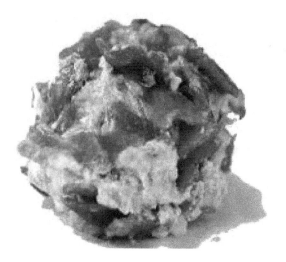

**Preparation Time**: 10 minutes

**Cooking Time:** 30 minutes

**Servings**: 6

**Ingredients Needed:**

- Bacon (about 4 oz. - 4 strips)

- Avocado (3.5 oz. or nearly half of 1 large)

- Small finely chopped chili pepper (1)

- Ghee or butter (.25 cup)

- Crushed cloves of garlic (2)

- Small minced onion (approximately 1.2 oz. or half of 1)

- Fresh lime juice (1 tbsp. or about .25 of a lime)

- Pinch of ground black pepper or cayenne (1 pinch)

- Salt (to your liking)

- Freshly chopped cilantro (1-2 tbsp.)

## Directions

1. Warm the oven temperature to reach 375° F.

2. Prepare a baking tray using a layer parchment baking paper.

3. Fry the bacon for 10 to 15 minutes. Save the grease for step five.

4. Peel, deseed, and chop the avocado into a dish along with the garlic, chili pepper, lime juice, cilantro, black pepper, salt, and butter. Use a fork or potato masher to combine the mixture. Blend in the onion.

5. Empty the grease into the bomb fixings, blend well, and cover for 20 to 30 minutes in the fridge.

6. Break up the bacon into a bowl and roll the six balls in it until coated evenly.

7. Serve when you want a delicious appetizer.

# Keto Salmon & Cream Cheese Bites

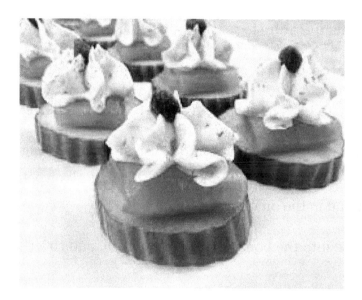

**Preparation Time**: 10 minutes

**Cooking Time:** 40 minutes

**Servings**: 6

**Ingredients Needed:**

- Salt (.5 tsp.)

- Cream or milk (1 cup)

- Eggs (6 medium)

- Dried dill (.5 tsp.)

- Cream cheese (.33 cup)

- Shredded cheese (.5 cup)

- Fresh/smoked salmon slices (1.8 oz.)

**Also Needed:** Mini muffin trays or silicone molds

## Preparation Method

1. Whisk the salt, eggs, and milk in a large measuring cup.

2. Fold in the smoked salmon, shredded cheese, and diced cream cheese.

3. Pour into the molds and bake for 10-15 minutes at 350° Fahrenheit.

4. Cool before removing to serve.

## Keto Summer Options

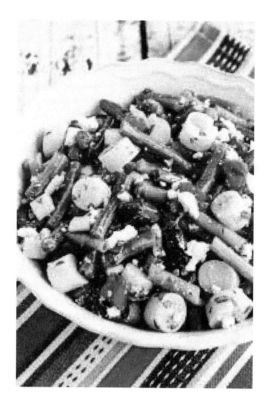

**Preparation Time**: 10 minutes

**Cooking Time**: 30 minutes

**Servings**: 6

**Ingredients Needed:**

- Cooked bacon (3 strips)

- Shredded cheddar cheese (1 cup)

**Directions**

1. Set the oven ahead of time to 350° F.

2. Prepare a baking tin with a sheet of parchment paper.

3. Pour about one tablespoon of the cheese onto the tray for each serving. Break the bacon to bits and add to the piles of cheese.

4. Bake for five to eight minutes and let cool. Blot the grease away with a paper towel before serving.

### a. Keto Coleslaw Stuffed Wraps

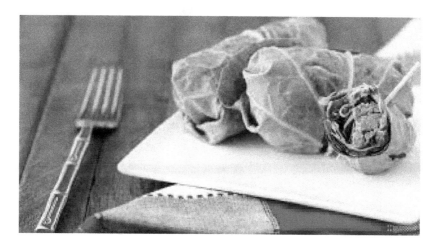

**Preparation Time**: 10 minutes

**Cooking Time**: 30 minutes

**Servings**: 6

**Ingredients Needed:**

- Sea salt (.25 tsp.)

- Green onions (.5 cup)

- Red cabbage (3 cups)

- Keto-friendly mayonnaise (.75 cup)

- Apple cider vinegar (2 tsp.) The Wraps & Other Fillings:

- Ground beef/turkey/pork/chicken– cooked & chilled (1 lb.)

- Collard leaves (16)

- Packed alfalfa sprouts (.33 cup)

- Toothpicks

## Directions

1.  Prepare the meat of choice in a frying pan. Thinly slice the cabbage. Remove the stems from the collards and dice the onions. Add all of the fixings in a large mixing container and stir well.

2.  Add a spoonful of the coleslaw on the far edge of the first collard leaf (the uncut side). Add the meat and the sprouts.

3.  Roll and tuck the sides and insert toothpicks at an angle to hold them together. Continue until all are done. Serve.

## Keto Dried Beef & Cream Cheese Ball

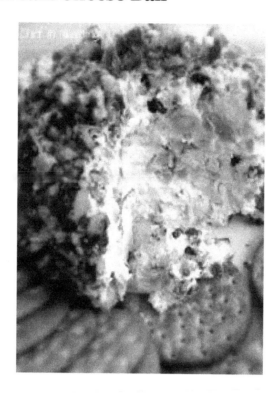

**Preparation Time**: 10 minutes

**Cooking Time**: 40 minutes

**Servings:** 6

**Ingredients Needed:**

- Shredded cheddar cheese (8 oz.)

- Cream cheese (3 oz.)

- Worcestershire sauce (.5 tsp.)

- Black olives (.25 cup)

- Salt (1 pinch of each): ○ Onion ○ Garlic ○ Celery

- Dried beef (4 oz. jar)

## Directions

1. Mince the dried beef and set it aside.

2. Combine the remainder of the fixings. Mix until smooth.

3. Shape the mixture into a ball and roll it through the beef.

4. Arrange them on a sheet of aluminum foil.

5. Refrigerate until you're ready to serve. Chill the ball overnight or for at least several hours.

# Keto Smoked Salmon Wraps

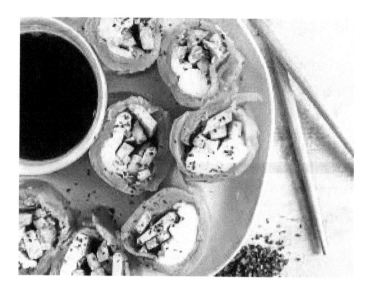

**Preparation Time**: 10 minutes

**Cooking Time**: 20 minutes

**Servings:** 6

**Ingredients Needed:**

- Coconut cream (1 tbsp.)

- Ham slices (4)

- Cucumber (half of 1)

- Smoked salmon (3.5 oz.)

- Green salad - for serving

**Directions**

1. Spread the coconut cream over each of the ham slices. Add a slice of smoked salmon.

2. For the next layer, add the thinly sliced pieces of cucumber.

3. Roll the fixings and place them on top of a fresh salad before serving.

# Fennel Quiche

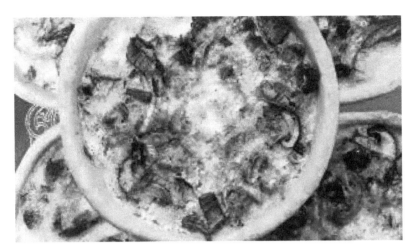

**Preparation Time**: 10 minutes

**Cooking Time**: 50 minutes

**Servings**: 6

**Ingredients:**

- oz. fennel, chopped

- 1 cup spinach

- eggs

- ½ cup almond flour

- 1 teaspoon olive oil

- 1 tablespoon butter

- 1 teaspoon salt

- ¼ cup heavy cream

- 1 teaspoon ground black pepper

## Directions:

1. Chop the spinach and combine it with the chopped fennel in the big bowl. Beat the egg in the separate bowl and whisk them.

2. Combine the whisked eggs with the almond flour, butter, salt, heavy cream, and ground black pepper. Whisk it.

3. Preheat the air fryer to 360 F. Spray the air fryer basket tray with the olive oil inside. Then add the spinach-fennel mixture and pour the whisked egg mixture.

4. Cook the quiche for 18 minutes. When the time is over – let the quiche chill little.

5. Then remove it from the air fryer and slice into the servings. Enjoy!

# Turkey Hash

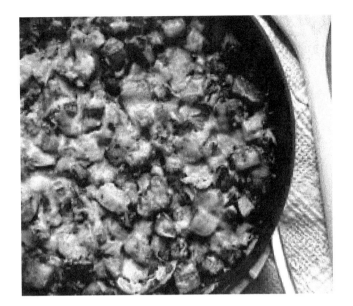

**Preparation Time:** 10 minutes

**Cooking Time:** 30 minutes

**Servings**: 6

**Ingredients**:

- cups cauliflower florets

- 1 small yellow onion, chopped

- Salt and ground black pepper, to taste

- 1/4 cup heavy cream

- 2 tbsp. unsalted butter

- 1 tsp. dried thyme

- 1-pound cooked turkey meat, chopped

## Directions:

1. In a pan of salted boiling water, add the cauliflower and cook for about 4 minutes. Drain the cauliflower well and rinse under cold running water.

2. Then chop the cauliflower and set aside. In a large skillet, melt the butter over medium heat and sauté onion for about 4-5 minutes.

3. Add thyme, salt and black pepper and sauté for about 1 minute. S

4. tir in cauliflower and cook for about 2 minutes. Stir in turkey and cook for about 5-6 minutes. Stir in the cream and cook for about 2 minutes more.

5. Serve warm.

# Lemon Salmon and Broccoli Casserole

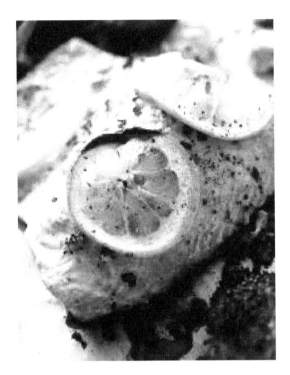

**Preparation Time:** 10 minutes

**Cooking Time:** 15 minutes

**Servings:** 4

**Ingredients:**

- 1 tablespoon of olive oil

- 1 onion finely chopped

- 1 cup of mushrooms

- 1 large broccoli

- 2 cloves garlic

- 1 lb smoked salmon

- 1 cup of cream

- 3/4 cup of water

- Lemon juices of 2 lemons

- Capers, to taste

- 1 cup of grated cheese

**Directions**:

1. Heat the olive oil in a large over-proof saucepan over medium heat and sauté the onions and mushrooms for 2 - 3 minutes.

2. Add the garlic and broccoli, cook, stirring occasionally, for a total of 5 minutes.

3. Add water and cream, and season with the salt and pepper.

4. Add the lemon juice and mix.

5. Add the cream, smoked salmon and capers and mix again.

6. Cover with the grated cheese and put in the oven, broil about 3 minutes, while the cheese is melted.

# Herbed Shrimp with Cilantro

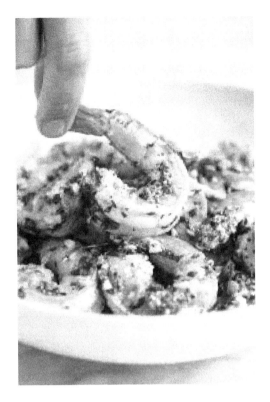

**Preparation Time:** 15 minutes

**Cooking Time:** 4 minutes

**Servings:** 4

**Ingredients:**

- 1 cup water

- 1 1/2 lb large shrimp, peeled

- 1 bunch cilantro, finely chopped

- 1/4 cup olive oil

- 1 cup grated tomato

- 2 cloves garlic, minced

- 1 teaspoon cumin

- 1 teaspoon coriander

- 1 teaspoon turmeric

- tablespoon of lime juice, freshly squeezed

**Directions:**

1  Pour water to the inner stainless-steel pot in the Instant Pot.

2  Add shrimp and sprinkle with chopped cilantro and pinch of salt.

3  In a bowl, stir together the olive oil, grated tomato, garlic, cumin, coriander, and turmeric.

4  Pour the mixture over shrimp and cilantro; toss to combine well.

5  Lock lid into place and set on the MANUAL setting for 3 -4 minutes.

6  When the timer beeps, press "Cancel" and carefully flip the Quick Release valve to let the pressure out.

7  Serve hot shrimp with sauce.

# CHAPTER 7:

# Most Common Keto Diet Mistakes

## Common Mistakes to Avoid on a Ketogenic Diet

### Not Getting Enough Magnesium, Potassium, and Sodium

Although usually, a regular diet contains plenty of sodium, because most processed food contains high amounts of salt, the majority of people do find that when they go keto and cut processed foods, they are low in it.

You may not think of low sodium as an issue, but this usually leads to fatigue and cravings.

Potassium is sometimes lacking more while you are on a ketogenic diet, so make sure you get enough of it, especially if you're an active person. Eating spinach and avocados can help you in this.

Lastly, magnesium is a mineral that many of us initially lack of. Many people point to the degradation of the soil as a possible explanation for our widespread shortcomings. Magnesium is essential for sleep, mood, muscles, and general well-being, so it is also good to ensure that you get enough of it. Drinking some bone broth is an excellent way to add more of these minerals to your ketogenic diet – it contains sodium, potassium, and magnesium.

## Not eating enough greens

The key to a ketogenic diet is eating fewer carbohydrates, and many people think that this means avoiding all vegetables.

Do not do that, please.

It's true that growing vegetables, such as onions or mushrooms, contain a reasonable amount of carbohydrates, so you may want to limit them, however, keeping eating a lot of vegetables is essential to ensure you get plenty of vitamins and minerals. There are several ways you can incorporate more vegetables into your diet. Salads, sauces, and green smoothies are all quick and easy to make.

Walking is one of the most natural options, but at home, you should also do bodyweight exercises such as push-ups, sit-ups, and squats.

## Running into Deficiencies in Salts and Minerals

The desire for sugars that is accused at the beginning can be exacerbated by a possible lack of minerals. It is therefore necessary to integrate with the right doses of potassium, magnesium, and sodium. Using Himalayan salt, eating salty snacks, using magnesium in the evening, could be just as many ways to remedy this mistake.

## Consume Too Much Protein

At the beginning, higher doses of protein help to overcome hunger crises, but then it is good to go back to consuming the right amount.

To find out how many proteins to consume, just multiply your body weight by 0.8 (if you make a normal physical effort) or 1.2 (if you are a sportsman).

Another common mistake is to consume poor quality proteins, such as pork and cold cuts.

## Insufficient Fat Consumption

This is another mistake that is easy to run into if we follow the ketogenic diet. We continue to be afraid of consuming fats and not using all-natural sources: coconut oil, ghee, MCT oil, egg yolk, fatty fish, butter, avocado. The opposite mistake is to exaggerate with oilseeds: walnuts, almonds, flax seeds, pumpkin seeds which, if we neglect to soak in advance with water and lemon, we also absorb the phytic acid they contain, a pro substance inflammatory and antinutrient.

## Consume Bad Quality Food

It is another of the most common mistakes. We focus on weight loss, but continue to consume frozen, canned, highly processed food and, as mentioned earlier, proteins that are practical and quick to eat but of poor quality.

## Do not Introduce the Right Amount of Fiber

Vegetables should always be fresh, consumed in twice the amount of protein and always cooked intelligently, that is, never subjected to overcooking or too high temperatures.

In everyday life, if present, however, we often resort to ready-made, frozen or packaged vegetables.

Also, with regard to fruit, we often resort to the very sugary one, we forget that there are many berries with a low glycemic index: berries, mulberries, goji berries, Inca berries, maqui.

## Eat Raw Vegetables

I know this may surprise you, but consuming large quantities of raw vegetables, centrifuged, cold smoothies, over time slow down digestion, cool it, undermine our ability to transform food and absorb nutrients. Over time, this exposes us to inevitable deficiencies: joint pain, teeth, nails and weak hair, anemia, tiredness, abnormal weight loss.

## Consume the Highest Protein Load at Dinner

This is a mistake that we all involuntarily tend to commit. The work, the thousand commitments, lead us to stay out all day, to eat a frugal meal for lunch or even not to consume it at all. Here the dinner turns into the only moment of the day in which we find our family members, we have more time, we are more relaxed, and we finally allow ourselves a real meal complete with vegetables, proteins, sometimes even carbohydrates and then fruit or dessert to finish.

It escapes us that even the healthiest protein, the freshest or most organic food, weighs down the liver. During the night, this being busy helping digestion, it cannot perform the other precious task: to purify the blood, prepare hormones, energy for the next day.

## <u>Not Drinking Enough</u>

And above all don't drink hot water. You got it right, drinking hot water is another story entirely, a huge difference from drinking it even at room temperature. The benefits are many: greater digestibility and absorption, deep hydration of cells, brighter skin and hair, retention disappears, cellulite improves, kidneys are strengthened, digestion improves, heartburn subsides.

# Food Supplements After 50

When you are first starting the Ketogenic Diet, I suggest trying it for a few weeks on your own. It is going to take some extra effort, but it is absolutely something you can do naturally. If you need a little boost, there are some supplements on the market that can help ease the transition.

Alpha Lipoic Acid and Chromium If you have issues with your insulin levels, Chromium and r-ALA may be able to help you out. While these two supplements claim to be insulin "mimickers," they actually help increase your sensitivity to insulin to help lower your insulin levels and heighten the glucagon. When this happens, you will get into ketosis quicker.

Hydroxymethylbutyrate (HMB) This is a popular ketogenic supplement known as BHB salt. It is used as a supplement to minimize the period before you get into ketosis, aka The Keto Flu. HMB is an exogenous ketone, meaning you will be putting synthetic ketone fuel into your body before it naturally makes the change itself. By doing this, it will make the transition time easier.

Carnitine You probably know this supplement as Acetyl L-Carnitine. This is a popular supplement to use as an energy booster. It seems now that L-Carnitine is actually needed to help boost the formation of ketones in the liver. When you take this supplement, it can help shift your metabolism from glycogen to ketones.

MCT Oil When you reach ketosis, MCT Oil can be extremely beneficial in keeping you there. This oil has high-quality fats that can give you a quick boost when you need it in your diet.

While this doesn't help make your transition more manageable, it will help once you are in ketosis.

Keto Multivitamin For any people starting a strict kept diet, it can become challenging to get all of your essential fiber, minerals, and vitamins. For this reason, you may want to consider a quality multivitamin. This will help provide you with minerals that are all lost as you transition into ketosis. Either way, you will want to consider taking a supplement that provides you with electrolytes to help you out during the transition process.

Fish Oil Finally, you will want to consider a supplement of fish oil. Remember that you will need to balance your omega-3s and omega-6s. While Americans generally get twenty times the amount of omega-6 fats they need, a fish oil or cod liver oil will be able to help you create that balance.

As you start aging, your body no longer functions the way it used to. Ideally, you should be able to get enough essential vitamins and nutrients from your diet but once you age, hormonal changes may lead to decreased functionality. Now's the time when you may need to start taking supplements in order to stay healthy. Here are a couple of vitamins and minerals you might need to add in your diet:

## **Vitamin D & Calcium**

Many older women become susceptible to bone loss as they age towards menopause. Thus, you may start to experience weaker joints as you hit your fifties. To cope with these deficiencies, you can add calcium and vitamin D supplements to your diet. Speak to your physician when deciding the dosage. The recommended amount is to split 1000mg of calcium for men and 1200mg for women into two doses. For calcium, you can consume more milk and yogurt, although keto advises that you don't go too crazy on the dairy.

Vitamin D is found in foods such as cod liver oil, fatty fish, and egg yolk, but in low quantities. The best choice is to take it directly thanks to the exposure of the body to the sun, but this is not always possible for everyone and all year round. The advice therefore is, when you are unable to expose yourself to the sun, so take vitamin D as a supplement. In general, the recommended daily amount is 2000 IU.

## Omega-3 Fatty Acids

Omega-3 fatty acids are an essential part of any diet and are known as 'good fats'. These fatty acids reduce inflammation, prevent irregular arteries, and keep your blood sugar levels in check. Some studies also indicate how it can also reduce the risks of Alzheimer's and heart disease.

This is why fish oil intake is so popular. These supplements contain large amounts of fatty acids. Fish oil is also known for improving skin texture by reducing dryness. It can also help lower triglycerides level in the body. Some healthy sources of omega-3 fatty acids include salmon and flaxseed oil.

## Probiotics

When you start getting old, you may experience gut-related issues. Probiotics include healthy bacteria that are good for your body. These organisms play an integral role in aiding digestion. Even younger folks are recommended to take probiotics to stay healthy.

Some natural food sources of probiotics include yogurt and kimchi.

## Vitamin B12

Vitamin B12 deficiency can lead to a number of problems including increased risks of dementia. However, it's also worth noting that too much of vitamin B12 can also lead to serious consequences. Speak to your doctor about including new supplements in your diet. Chances are if you're eating right, you might not need any supplements at all.

Healthy food sources of vitamin B12 include trout and clams.

Staying healthy requires engaging in a number of physical and mental activities to stay active. But eating healthy using supplements when necessary is also an important part of happy living. Most of these supplements can be taken orally but you can also purchase swallowing pills. Regardless of what you opt for, be sure to check with your doctor.

## Precautions to Take Before Starting on Supplements

Dietary supplements are not to be taken lightly. Here are a couple of precautions you should take before adding it to your diet: Speak to your doctor

We can't stress about this enough. Even if you're opting for organic supplements, it's important that you consult a doctor. Taking supplements with certain medication can sometimes lead to side effects and dangerous chemical reactions. This becomes especially important if you suffer from allergies or are already on some kind of medication for a health ailment. Whenever possible, try to persuade your doctor into recommending a natural supplement.

## Understand That Supplements Don't Substitute Nutrition

It's important to understand that these supplements are not a replacement for proper nutrition. It's still essential to eat a healthy diet. Following a healthy keto diet should get you plenty of nutrients if you're eating the right foods. Supplements are only there to help fill the gap in case you're not able to get all of your vitamins and minerals right.

We urge you to consume a nutrient rich diet and not one that this full of unhealthy fats.

## Research before Joining the Club

One of the most authentic ways to compare supplement brands is to check ratings online. You can also seek help from friends and family to find out what brands they trust in. We urge you to check for certifications that indicate that the product is GMP, Organic, and Vegan etc. Unfortunately, there are a number of ineffective supplements out there that fail to help the consumer in any way.

## Consider Your Options

Nobody knows you better than yourself! If you suffer from allergies or have an experience of digestive issues, thoroughly read through the ingredients. Note that capsules are easier to consume and can be easier to swallow when compared to solid tablets.

Ingredients such as ginger and chamomile also have soothing effects that ease stomach and mouth problems. Only include supplements in your diet that are safe to consume and won't result in any dangerous side effects. You also want to stick to supplements that you can easily consume every day.

## Seek Professional Help

Most online stores or even regular stores have expert nutritionists on board who would be happy to guide you. You can reach out for a professional consultation online where all you have to do is enter a couple of details. Most of these consultations are free and are offered as a promotion. Make sure to ask questions about any ingredients that you've been second guessing about.

## Know the Manufacturer

We urge you to steer clear from excessively cheap products. These products are often made using low quality ingredients which can potentially lead to a number of side effects and health problems. When it comes to your health, only opt for reliable brands and manufacturers who have been in the business for several years. You should also opt for manufacturers and companies who prioritize customer satisfaction.

# Conversion and Replacements Tables

## Equivalents

| U.S. | U.S. |
|---|---|
| 16 tablespoons | 1 cup |
| 12 tablespoons | 3/4 cup |
| 10 tablespoons + 2 teaspoons | 2/3 cup |
| 8 tablespoons | 1/2 cup |
| 6 tablespoons | 3/8 cup |
| 5 tablespoons + 1 teaspoons | 1/3 cup |
| 4 tablespoons | 1/4 cup |
| 2 tablespoons + 2 teaspoons | 1/6 cup |
| 2 tablespoons | 1/8 cup |
| 1 tablespoon | 1/16 cup |
| 1 pint | 2 cups |
| 1 quart | 2 pints |
| 1 tablespoon | 3 teaspoons |
| 1 cup | 48 teaspoons |
| 1 cup | 16 tablespoons |

## Capacity

| U.S. | METRIC |
|---|---|

| | |
|---|---|
| 1/5 teaspoon | 1 ml |
| 1 teaspoon (tsp) | 5 ml |
| 1 tablespoon (tbsp) | 15 ml |
| 1 fluid oz. | 30 ml |
| 1/5 cup | 50 ml |
| 1/4 cup | 60 ml |
| 1/3 cup | 80 ml |
| 3.4 fluid oz. | 100 ml |
| 1/2 cup | 120 ml |
| 2/3 cup | 160 ml |
| 3/4 cup | 180 ml |
| 1 cup | 240 ml |
| 1 pint (2 cups) | 480 ml |
| 1 quart (4 cups) | .95 liter |
| 34 fluid oz. | 1 liter |
| 4.2 cups | 1 liter |
| 2.1 pints | 1 liter |
| 1.06 quarts | 1 liter |
| .26 gallon | 1 liter |
| 4 quarts (1 gallon) | 3.8 liters |

# Weight

| U.S. | METRIC |
|---|---|

| | |
|---|---|
| .035 ounce | 1 gram |
| 0.5 oz. | 14 grams |
| 1 oz. | 28 grams |
| 1/4 pound (lb) | 113 grams |
| 1/3 pound (lb) | 151 grams |
| 1/2 pound (lb) | 227 grams |
| 1 pound (lb) | 454 grams |
| 1.10 pounds (lbs.) | 500 grams |
| 2.205 pounds (lbs.) | 1 kilogram |
| 35 oz. | 1 kilogram |

# Conclusion

Assuming that it does not go through the negative effects of healthcare difficulties, a keto diet can offer many benefits, especially to reduce weight loss. Basically, eating whole food is probably the most effective way to eat intensely, basically because it is a supportive strategy.

It is important to note that many studies show that ketogenic weight loss is really difficult to maintain. Therefore, the best advice is to find a consistent way of eating that suits you.

By having a clear understanding of what you should be eating and how you should be feeling, you can compare the way that you feel to the way that the diet is supposed to make you feel. This allows you to stay in control of your diet without feeling that you have to completely surrender all of your decision-making.

We all have our own bad habits, and a lot of us have bad eating habits. In today's society, it becomes easy to fall into these habits because of the promise of convenience. If you had the choice to get takeout or make a meal for yourself in a hurry, you would likely opt for takeout because you have been trained to believe that it is faster and easier. While it might be faster, you are likely compromising the quality of the food that you are eating because it appears more convenient. Most of the time, it doesn't take that much additional effort to cook for yourself. With the way that society pushes fast food and various food delivery services, it is no wonder that you would be more comfortable with allowing someone else to make your food.

While some of these services can be incredibly convenient, you are settling yourself short because you do not know exactly what you are eating. You do not know where the ingredients are from and how they were prepared. These things matter to your overall health, especially as aging becomes a factor. More than ever, you need to be paying attention to the source of your food. When you let these decisions go out of your control, you are allowing others to decide what is best for your body. Even when you begin to feel sluggish and less functional, the body becomes easily addicted to junk food so it will trick you into thinking that you need to keep eating this way.

The trick is to find your balance, one step at a time if you must, as long as you are working to your end goal. How long it takes to get you there is entirely up to you. Don't think you have to rush headlong into it. Set achievable realistic goals that you feel one hundred percent comfortable with, otherwise your intermittent fasting diet is not going to work.

This is a lifestyle change, not a fad diet that you try for a few days or weeks and then forget because it became mundane or too challenging. This is a diet and lifestyle you need to commit to that will not only help you lose weight but be beneficial for your health. There is nothing wrong with easing into it; it is not a race and you have to remember you are doing this for you!

The Keto food plan is a low-carb diet that is designed to place the human frame into a heightened Ketogenic state, which might inevitably result in higher pronounced fat burn and weight loss. It is a reasonably accessible food regimen with a variety of keto-friendly meals being readily available in marketplaces at highly low prices. It isn't an eating regimen that is reserved most effectively for the affluent and elite.

As some distance as effectiveness is concerned, there's just no denying how impactful a keto eating regimen maybe for someone who wants to lose a drastic quantity of weight in a wholesome and managed manner. The keto weight-reduction plan also enforces discipline and precision for the agent by incorporating macro counting and meal journaling to ensure accuracy and accountability in the weight-reduction project. There are no external factors that can impact how robust this weight loss plan may be for you. Everything is within your control.

And lastly, it's a reasonably sustainable weight loss plan, for the reason that it doesn't compromise on taste or range. Sure, there are lots of restrictions. But ultimately, there are lots of alternatives and workarounds that can assist stave off cravings. If these kinds of standards and reasons are observed in your personal life, then it could genuinely be safe to say that the Keto food plan is a high-quality one for you.

CPSIA information can be obtained
at www.ICGtesting.com
Printed in the USA
LVHW060000111220
673819LV00030B/1226